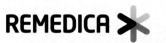

The PVAC® Workbook

Techniques to Map and Ablate Atrial Fibrillation

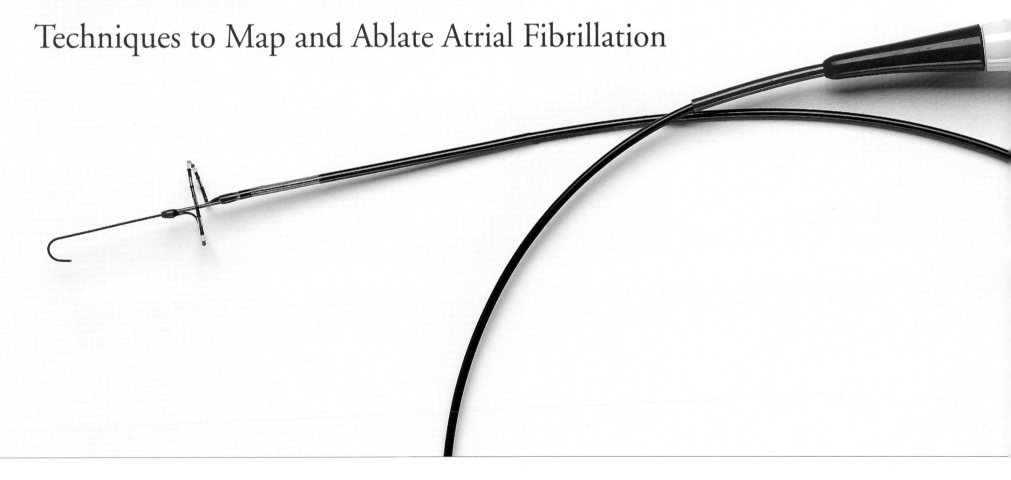

Published by Remedica

Commonwealth House, 1 New Oxford Street, London, WC1A 1NU, UK
Willis Tower, 233 S Wacker Drive, Suite 3425, Chicago, IL 60606, USA
books@remedica.com
www.remedica.com
Tel: +44 (0)20 7759 2999
Fax: +44 (0)20 7759 2951

Publisher: Andrew Ward

In-house editors: James Griffin, Leonard Wills
Commissioning editor: Charlotte Palmer
Design and Artwork: AS&K Skylight Creative Services

Remedica is a member of the AS&K Media Partnership.

ISBN: 978-1-905721-58-0

British Library Cataloguing-in-Publication Data.
A catalogue record for this book is available from the British Library.

Printed in Hungary

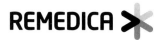

The PVAC® Workbook

Techniques to Map and Ablate Atrial Fibrillation

Lucas Boersma, Mattias Duytschaever, J. Christoph Geller, Christoph Scharf

Lucas Boersma, MD, PhD
Cardiology Department
St Antonius Hospital Nieuwegein
Nieuwegein
The Netherlands

Mattias Duytschaever, MD, PhD
Department of Cardiology
St Jan Hospital Bruges
Bruges
Belgium

J. Christoph Geller, MD
Zentralklinik Bad Berka
Bad Berka
Germany

Christoph Scharf, MD
Internal Medicine and Cardiology
Cardiovascular Center
Im Park Clinic
Zurich
Switzerland

Biographies

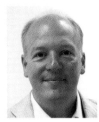

Lucas Boersma, MD, PhD

Lucas Boersma was born in Heerlen, The Netherlands, in 1965. He received his medical degree from Maastricht University in 1994. During his medical training he became involved in experimental electrophysiology at Maastricht University, under the supervision of Professor Maurits Allessie, working with animal models on the project "Ventricular tachycardia in the rabbit heart" for which he received a PhD degree in 1994 and the "Hamburger Award 1995" from the Dutch Society for Physiology. In 2000, he finished his cardiology training at St Antonius Hospital, Nieuwegein, The Netherlands (supervised by Professor Norbert van Hemel). He then relocated to the Hospital Clinic of Barcelona, Spain, for his clinical electrophysiology training in 2001 (supervised by Professor Josep Brugada), which

was supported by a fellowship award from the European Society of Cardiology. Since 2002, he has been a member of the Cardiology Department of St Antonius Hospital, Nieuwegein, working as a clinical electrophysiologist. In 2006 Dr Boersma became involved with the first experimental work with multielectrode catheters and phased radiofrequency energy in patients, and subsequently participated in animal studies and in all the clinical trials from Ablation Frontiers, Inc. He was the first to publish clinical results with this new technology. To date, there have been more than 550 cases of multielectrode ablation performed at St Antonius Hospital, Nieuwegein. Dr Boersma is a proctor and trainer for multielectrode ablation of atrial fibrillation.

Dr Boersma would like to acknowledge Maurits Wijffels, MD, PhD and Eric Wever, MD, PhD, both of whom are cardiology staff members at St Antonius Hospital, Nieuwegein.

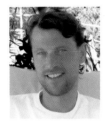

Mattias Duytschaever, MD, PhD

Mattias Duytschaever was born in Ghent, Belgium, in 1970. He obtained his medical degree in 1995 from the University of Ghent, after which he conducted research for his PhD into the role of atrial electrical remodeling in the management of atrial fibrillation until 2000, under the supervision of Professor Maurits Allessie, at Maastricht University, The Netherlands. Professor Duytschaever furthered his training in cardiology at the Academic Hospital Ghent, Belgium, from 2000 to 2002, and became Professor in Electrophysiology at the University of Ghent in 2003. Since 2006, he has conducted diagnostic and interventional electrophysiology at the Department of Electrophysiology at St Jan Hospital Bruges, Belgium, while still providing his services as Professor in Electrophysiology at the University of Ghent. Professor Duytschaever is an active clinical researcher at both of these establishments and has published widely on the pathogenesis and treatment of arrhythmias. He is a reviewer for *Lancet*, the *European Heart Journal*, *Europace*, and the *Journal of Cardiovascular Electrophysiology*. In 2010, Professor Duytschaever was selected as Principal Investigator to an international, randomized, multicenter study on catheter ablation of atrial fibrillation.

Professor Duytschaever would like to acknowledge Yves Vandekerckhove, MD, Rene Tavernier, MD, PhD, and Richard Houben, PhD from St Jan Hospital Bruges for their contribution and interpretation of the electrogram tracings.

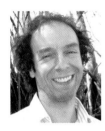

J. Christoph Geller, MD

J. Christoph Geller was born in 1959 in Bonn, Germany, and attended medical school at the University of Bonn and Basel, Switzerland. He completed an internship and residency training in internal medicine and a Fellowship in Cardiology at University Hospitals in Bonn, Germany. After a post-doctoral research fellowship at the Department of Pharmacology at Columbia University, New York, NY, USA from 1991 to 1993, he attended University Hospitals in Cleveland, OH, USA from 1993 to 1995 where he completed a fellowship in clinical electrophysiology. Dr Geller was the attending physician and Director of the Arrhythmia Service at the Division of Cardiology, at University Hospitals in Magdeburg, Germany from 1995 to 2004. Since 2004, he has been the Chief of the Arrhythmia Section, Division of Cardiology, Zentralklinik Bad Berka, Germany, and since 2007 he has been Professor of Medicine at the Otto-von-Guericke University in Magdeburg. His areas of interest and research include nonpharmacological treatment of cardiac arrhythmias using catheter ablation and implantable devices.

Dr Geller would like to acknowledge Santi Raffa, MD, PhD, Michele Brunelli, MD, and Anett Grosse, MD, who are actively involved with PVAC at Zentralklinik Bad Berka.

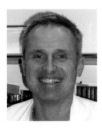

Christoph Scharf, MD

Christoph Scharf was born in 1966 and attended medical school in Zurich and Paris between 1985 and 1991. He undertook residencies in anesthesia from 1992 to 1994, in internal medicine from 1994 to 1996, in tropical medicine in Chad, Africa in 1996/1997, and in internal medicine between 1997 and 1999. Dr Scharf received board certification in internal medicine (FMH). Between 1999 and 2001 he started cardiology fellowship training in Zurich, and in 2001/2002 achieved an electrophysiology fellowship at the University of Michigan, Ann Arbor, MI, USA, followed by a second year as staff physician in 2002/2003. On returning to the University Hospital Zurich he completed cardiology board examinations (FMH) and obtained the Venia legendi (Habilitation) at the University of Zurich for clinical cardiac electrophysiology. Since 2005, Dr Scharf has worked in private practice at Im Park Clinic, Zurich, the largest electrophysiology center in Switzerland. In 2006, he led the first multicenter trial that used duty-cycled radiofrequency ablation, and since then has been a regular proctor and trainer in clinical mentoring courses in atrial fibrillation ablation.

Dr Scharf would like to acknowledge Lam Dang, MSc, PhD, who is a signal processing engineer at Im Park Clinic, Zurich.

Contents

Foreword

Atrial fibrillation (AF) has become one of the most frequently targeted conditions of ablationists in recent years. The cornerstone of AF ablation is pulmonary vein isolation, and as new technologies that facilitate this process are developed, the number of electrophysiologists who perform AF ablation procedures will undoubtedly increase. The Pulmonary Vein Ablation Catheter® (PVAC®), a multielectrode catheter that allows the delivery of radiofrequency energy at multiple electrodes simultaneously, is an example of one such state-of-the-art technology. This book, *The PVAC® Workbook: Techniques to Map and Ablate Atrial Fibrillation*, will prove to be an invaluable resource both for electrophysiologists who are just beginning to ablate AF in the electrophysiology laboratory, and for experienced ablationists who are not yet fully skilled in the use of the PVAC. The authors have succeeded admirably in creating a workbook that is easy to comprehend and elucidative, and that focuses on information that is of practical value in the electrophysiology laboratory. The schematic drawings, fluoroscopic images, and intracardiac tracings will greatly enhance the ability of the reader to translate the knowledge presented in this workbook into clinical practice. Much of the detail, such as how to direct the catheter to each of the four pulmonary veins, is specific to the PVAC. However, the chapters on fluoroscopic topography of the pulmonary veins, confirmation of pulmonary vein isolation, differential pacing techniques, and adenosine challenge are generic in nature and should prove very helpful to trainees and electrophysiologists not yet familiar with AF ablation, regardless of the ablation technology being used.

Drs Boersma, Duytschaever, Geller, and Scharf have created an elegant and deceptively straightforward compendium of everything that the operator needs to know for isolating pulmonary veins with the PVAC. In the end, the individuals who will benefit most from their efforts are the countless patients with symptomatic AF whose quality of life can be enhanced by catheter ablation.

Fred Morady, MD
University of Michigan Medical Center
Ann Arbor, MI, USA

Acknowledgments

The authors would like to acknowledge Alessandro Dulio, BS, and Valerio Misiti, BS, for their support. Without their continued enthusiasm, this project would never have been possible. The authors would also like to acknowledge Juliet Percival for her wonderful device and anatomical illustrations that have added great value to the book, and thank Remedica and AS&K Skylight Creative Services for their editorial support and design and layout expertise.

1 | From Generator to Pulmonary Vein Isolation

This chapter describes the Pulmonary Vein Ablation Catheter® (PVAC®; Medtronic Ablation Frontiers, LLC, Carlsbad, CA, USA) and the ablation system, how it compares with conventional-tip ablation catheters, and the electrode design that enables the required current density to be achieved with less power compared with conventional catheters. The benefits of duty-cycling and the use of phasing to deliver a mixture of unipolar and bipolar energy are also illustrated. Finally, lesion characterization while using this catheter is elucidated as is the interpretation of temperature and power readings.

Learning Objectives

> *To understand the biophysics of delivering radiofrequency energy via a nonirrigated, multielectrode catheter*

> *To understand the concept of "duty-cycled" delivery of "phased radiofrequency energy"*

> *To comprehend the concept of unipolar and bipolar radiofrequency energy*

Introduction

The current concepts for catheter ablation of atrial fibrillation (AF), the most common cardiac arrhythmia, are based on the seminal work by Michel Haïssaguerre and colleagues. Initiation of AF is often the result of frequent atrial premature beats, originating in the left atrium close to the orifice of one of the four pulmonary veins (PVs). Therefore, isolation of the PVs is now the cornerstone of most ablation strategies used in patients with AF.

Conventional radiofrequency (RF) energy catheters with tip electrodes of 4 to 8 mm are not ideal for linear ablation in this complex anatomical area. This means that sophisticated supporting technology, such as three-dimensional mapping, is required to navigate these "two-dimensional catheters."

To overcome these limitations, attempts have been made in recent years to develop specific catheter designs that are better suited to the complex target area of the PV ostium, obviating the need for mapping systems. Hence, the emergence of the "three-dimensional catheters."

One of these new catheters, the PVAC, is the topic of this book. An advantage of this particular catheter is that each electrode pair can be used for mapping before ablation, the ablation itself, validation of vein isolation, and for pacing.

The PVAC and the Ablation System

The catheter

The PVAC is a 10-pole circular catheter capable of both mapping and ablation. It consists of a 9-F, 10-electrode, over-the-wire deflectable catheter with a 25-mm diameter spiral array at the distal end (**Figure 1**).

A new multichannel ablation generator (GENius™ Radiofrequency Generator, Medtronic Ablation Frontiers, LLC, Carlsbad, CA, USA) allows unipolar and bipolar ablation energy to be delivered independently to any of the electrodes in a temperature-controlled manner. For bipolar energy delivery, the electrodes are used in pairs. Energy can be delivered either to all five pairs or to a selection of electrode pairs. In addition, stimulation from all of the electrodes is possible, enabling the catheter to be used to confirm exit block after energy application.

Figure 1. The Pulmonary Vein Ablation Catheter (PVAC).

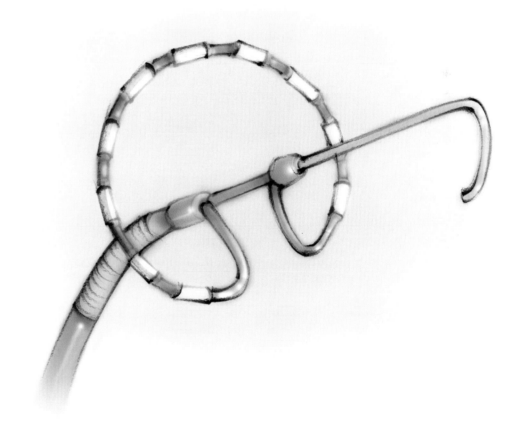

Positioning the catheter in the pulmonary vein

The catheter is positioned at the ostium of the PV over a conventional guidewire. By selecting individual vein side branches, contact with the chamber wall can be optimized (**Figure 2**).

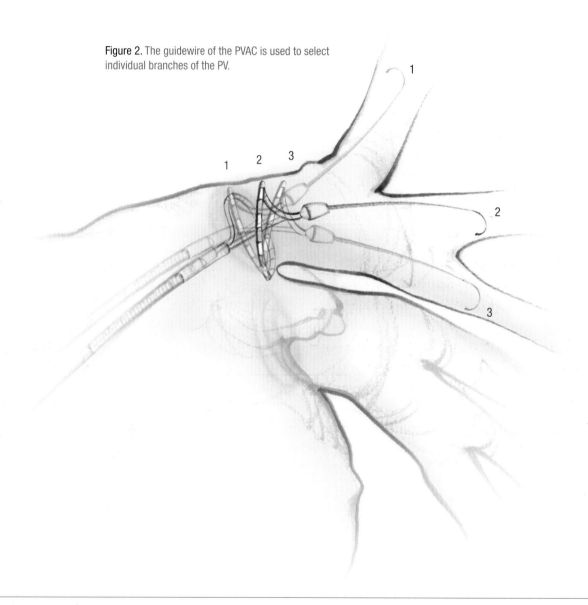

Figure 2. The guidewire of the PVAC is used to select individual branches of the PV.

Special electrode design and benefits for energy delivery

With the PVAC, RF energy is delivered in a temperature-controlled manner via a generator that has a maximum power limit of 10 W. Each cylindrical 3-mm electrode has a unique distal thermocouple (shown in blue) that, by design, is orientated towards the electrode–tissue interface. This allows: (i) accurate measurement of the temperature at the electrode–tissue interface, (ii) adjustable power modulation for each individual electrode, and (iii) maintenance of tissue temperature within a desirable temperature range.

Electrode cooling is achieved without active irrigation and is based upon: (i) "duty-cycled" RF current delivery allowing cooling during "off" periods (*see later*) and (ii) passive circulatory cooling resulting from blood flow (**Figure 3**).

Figure 3. PVAC electrode cooling is achieved as a result of the specially designed shape of the electrode.

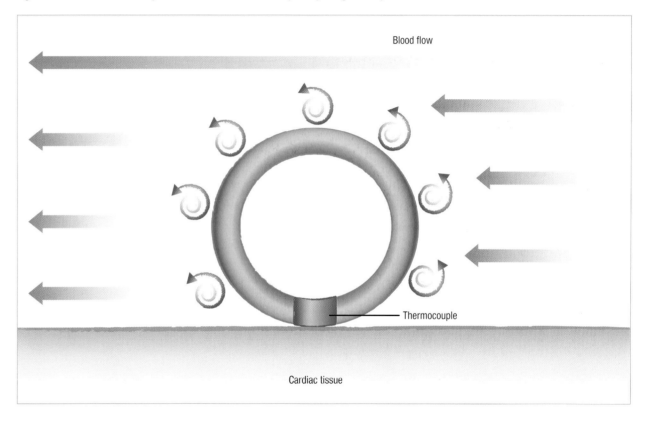

Blood flow

Thermocouple

Cardiac tissue

Comparison with conventional-tip catheters

In the PVAC, the array of multiple small electrodes can have power output adjusted at each electrode in order to achieve a target temperature. This alleviates thermal gradients, "hot spots", or overheating, which can occur on using single large electrodes (**Figure 4**).

In **Figure 4a**, a conventional ablation catheter with a 4-mm tip is shown. As a consequence of the variable orientation of the electrode tip and the resulting angle at the electrode–tissue interface, the temperature reading may not accurately reflect that of the tissue, leading to potential large differences in tissue temperature and hot spots (shown in red at the distal margins of the lesion forming under the electrode).

This is in contrast with the arrangement of electrodes in the newly designed PVAC. The thermocouple for each electrode is situated directly at the electrode–tissue interface, which creates a sort of long "virtual electrode" and allows a more precise, local temperature measurement to be made. This leads to a lower likelihood of temperature gradients or overheating (**Figure 4b**). In addition, the array of small electrodes, each of which measures local tissue temperature, brings about a more uniform temperature across the entire lesion, with less overheating compared with larger electrodes.

Figure 4. Thermal gradients and hot spots observed with (a) conventional ablation catheters are alleviated with (b) the "virtual electrode" of the PVAC.

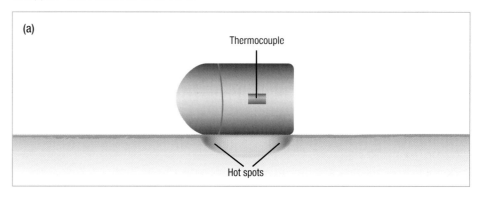

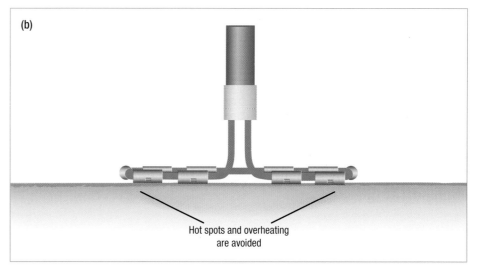

Relationship between electrode size and current density

Lesion formation by RF energy is governed by current density rather than total current. Current density is defined as the current per square millimeter (A/mm^2).

On using a conventional ablation catheter with a 4-mm tip, a power of 30 W results in a current density of approximately 0.017 A/mm^2 (**Figure 5a**).

In contrast, because of the smaller electrode size (3 mm) of the PVAC, less power (10 W) is needed to achieve comparable current density (**Figure 5b**) and lesions.

Figure 5. Comparison of current density between **(a)** conventional ablation catheters and **(b)** the PVAC.

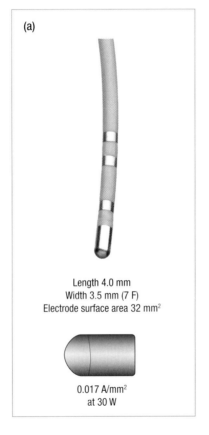

(a)

Length 4.0 mm
Width 3.5 mm (7 F)
Electrode surface area 32 mm^2

0.017 A/mm^2
at 30 W

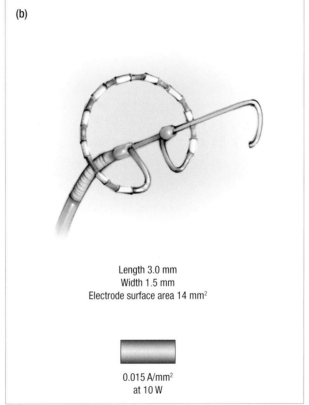

(b)

Length 3.0 mm
Width 1.5 mm
Electrode surface area 14 mm^2

0.015 A/mm^2
at 10 W

Duty-cycled energy delivery

The generator delivers 100 W peak in a duty-cycled mode. The term "duty cycle" describes a period of "on" and "off" time. RF energy is delivered only during the "on" period, which has a maximum duration of 10% of the cycle. Thus, the averaged RF energy (area-under-the-curve or root-mean-square [RMS]) delivered during PVAC ablation has a maximum value of 10 W (**Figure 6**).

Power modulation is needed to achieve and maintain the target temperature at the electrode–tissue interface. Power modulation in the system is regulated by altering the length of the "on" portion of the duty cycle. If less power is needed to achieve the target temperature, then the "on" period will be shortened. For example, 8 W is delivered by shortening the "on" period to 8%.

The "off" time in between RF energy delivery (by design ≥90% of the time) allows the electrodes to cool, enabling more power to be delivered into the tissue.

Figure 6. Sample of RF energy delivered during PVAC ablation.

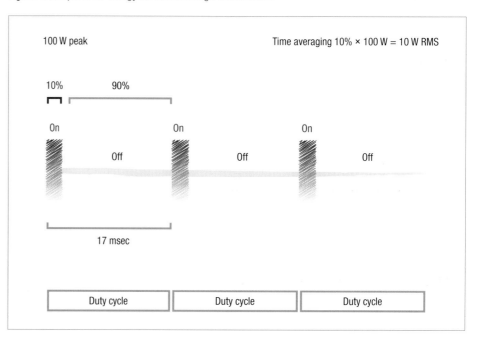

Unipolar and bipolar energy delivery: phasing

The generator can deliver power to each electrode individually, enabling control of both amplitude and phase. In order to deliver a mixture of unipolar and bipolar energy, the system utilizes a feature called *phasing*. If an electrode pair is *in phase*, there is no difference between the voltage of the pair and so current only flows to the "indifferent" (reference) electrode, meaning that power is delivered in a *unipolar manner* only. If an electrode pair is *out of phase*, there is still unipolar current, but in addition, there is also current flowing in a *bipolar manner* between the electrodes because of the voltage difference between them. This is explained in **Figures 7** and **8**.

In phase

In **Figure 7** the sinusoidal waves depict voltage. The red wave is the voltage at electrode 1, the blue wave is the voltage at electrode 2. There is no voltage difference between the electrodes at any moment in time—thus there is no current flow between both poles (no bipolar energy). As the voltage oscillates between positive and negative peaks, the current moves to and from the ablation electrodes and the return electrodes that are situated at the back of the patient (unipolar energy delivery).

Figure 7. Unipolar energy delivery. If an electrode pair is in phase (red and blue waves of electrodes 1 and 2, respectively), there is no difference between the voltage of the pair, and so current only flows to the "indifferent" (reference) electrode (unipolar only).

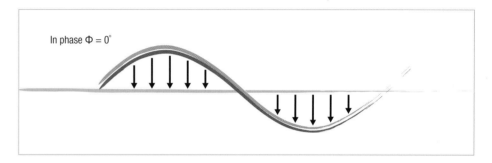

In phase Φ = 0˚

Out of phase

If the voltages for electrodes 1 and 2 move out of phase by 180°, a voltage difference is created between electrodes 1 and 2 (**Figure 8**). This difference in voltage drives bipolar energy delivery. When electrode 1 is at its positive peak, electrode 2 is at its negative nadir, and current will flow down from electrode 1 to electrode 2—in addition to flowing from electrode 1 to the return electrode. When electrode 2 is at its positive peak, electrode 1 is at its negative nadir. Thus, current will flow down from electrode 2 to electrode 1—in addition to flowing from electrode 2 to the return electrode. In this situation, there is both unipolar and bipolar energy delivery.

Figure 8. Bipolar and unipolar energy delivery. If an electrode pair is out of phase 180° (red and blue waves of electrodes 1 and 2, respectively), a voltage difference is created between electrodes 1 and 2 which drives bipolar in addition to unipolar energy delivery. Thus, current will flow between electrodes 1 and 2 in addition to flowing from both electrodes to the return electrode. Comparing bipolar and unipolar voltages, the bipolar voltage (↕) is twice that of unipolar voltage ($V_{Bipolar} = 2*V_{Unipolar}$). Given the equation $P = V^2/R$, bipolar power is four-fold greater than unipolar power.

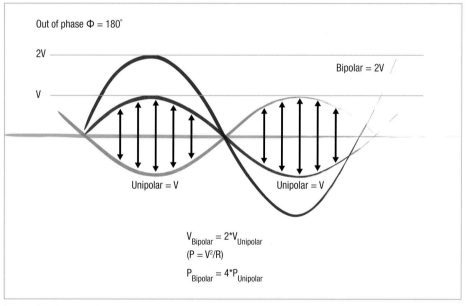

Out of phase Φ = 180°

2V

V

Bipolar = 2V

Unipolar = V   Unipolar = V

$$V_{Bipolar} = 2*V_{Unipolar}$$
$$(P = V^2/R)$$
$$P_{Bipolar} = 4*P_{Unipolar}$$

P: power; R: resistance; V: voltage.

Figure 9 shows that when power delivery is in phase there is only a voltage difference between the electrodes and the indifferent electrode (white field, ↕), but not between electrodes 1 and 2. In contrast, when power is delivered out of phase, in addition to the voltage difference between the electrodes and the indifferent electrode, there is also a voltage difference between electrodes 1 and 2 (yellow field, ↔).

Figure 9. Summary of (a) unipolar (in-phase) and (b) bipolar and unipolar (out-of-phase) energy delivery.

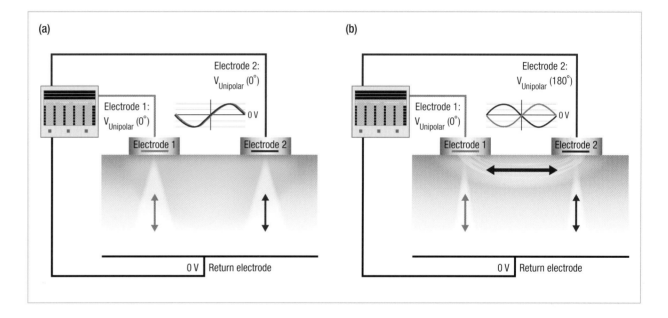

Sequential fields

In order to provide different energy modes with varying mixtures of unipolar and bipolar energy the generator uses a construct called "fields". The energy delivery is broken down into eight "sequential fields", but for illustrative purposes only the first four representative fields of each construct are shown.

During the "on" period of these fields, RF energy can be delivered either out of phase or in phase. When out-of-phase RF energy is delivered during each consecutive field, it is done so in a 16:4 or 4:1 ratio (**Figure 10a**). This implies that in a 4:1 generator setting, 80% of RF energy is delivered in the bipolar mode whereas 20% is delivered in the unipolar mode.

When out-of-phase RF energy is delivered during only two fields, with in-phase RF energy delivered during the other two fields, RF energy is delivered in an 8:4 or 2:1 ratio (**Figure 10b**). This implies that in a 2:1 generator setting, 66.6% of RF energy is delivered in the bipolar mode, whereas 33.3% is delivered in the unipolar mode.

When out-of-phase RF energy is delivered during only one field, with in-phase RF energy delivered during the other three fields, RF energy is delivered in a 4:1 or 1:1 ratio (**Figure 10c**). This implies that in a 1:1 generator setting, 50% of RF energy is delivered in the bipolar mode and 50% is delivered in the unipolar mode.

Figure 10. Examples of sequential fields used to modulate power into three different ratios. **(a)** Out-of-phase RF energy delivery in a 4:1 ratio, **(b)** an equal number of out-of-phase and in-phase RF energy fields leads to a delivery ratio of 2:1, and **(c)** out-of-phase RF energy delivery in a 1:1 ratio.

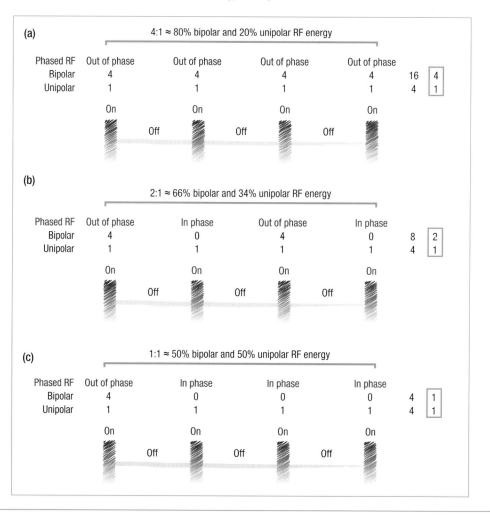

Lesion depth can be adjusted by varying the mixture of unipolar and bipolar energy. Unipolar delivery occurs from the ablation electrode to the return electrode and drives lesion depth; bipolar delivery occurs between adjacent ablation electrodes and is intended to close the gaps between adjacent electrodes ("fill") (**Figure 11**). The ability to control lesion depth by varying the ratio of unipolar to bipolar energy delivery may help to minimize damage to the surrounding tissue (eg, esophagus, phrenic nerve).

Figure 11. Lesion depth can be adjusted by varying the mixture of unipolar and bipolar energy.

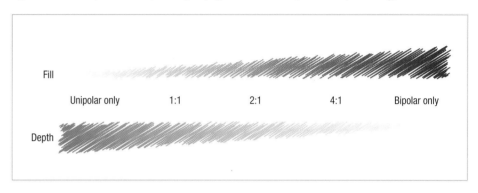

In vitro lesion characterization using the PVAC

Figure 12 shows the decrease in lesion depth from unipolar to bipolar energy (application) modes in an *in vitro* experimental scenario. The results demonstrate that the lesion depth increases in a controlled manner with increasing unipolar energy. This feature of the generator can be used to titrate lesion depth during PV isolation.

In circumstances where 4:1 RF energy delivery cannot isolate the PVs (eg, as on the ridge of the left-sided veins), then a ratio with a higher unipolar component may be considered (eg, 2:1).

In contrast, at the posterior wall of the left atrium and in areas within close proximity of critical structures in the surrounding tissue, lesions should be limited to the energy modes with a higher ratio of bipolar energy (eg, 4:1) in order to avoid deep penetration of the energy into the tissue.

Figure 12. *In vitro* experiment showing an increasing lesion depth with increasing unipolar energy on using the PVAC.

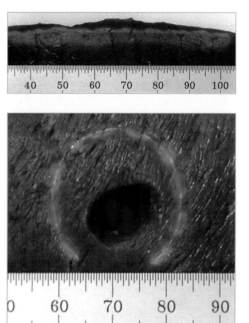

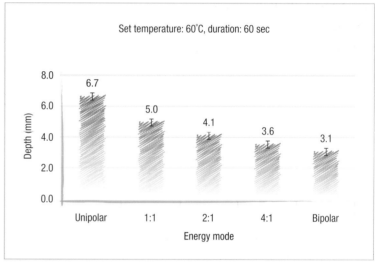

How to Interpret Temperature and Power Readings

Since RF energy is used for lesion generation, good contact with the wall of the ostium is required for optimal lesion formation and to minimize the risk of complications (eg, thrombus formation and "steam pops"). The generator screen can help to assess whether or not the catheter is in good contact with the atrial wall.

Thus, it is important to consider both the delivered power and the interface temperature. The temperature results from power output and cooling. It is color-coded in green if within 5°C of the target temperature (ie, >55°C), in blue if <55°C, in yellow if >5°C above the target temperature, or in red if >70°C.

Figure 13 shows an example on the generator screen of good catheter contact during 4:1 ablation. Note that all 10 of the columns (representing the five electrode pairs) are green and that the delivered power is ≥6 W for each column. In addition to the color of the columns, the total time that each electrode is within its target range for temperature is shown at the bottom of each column.

Figure 13. An example of good catheter contact in the ostium during 4:1 ablation.

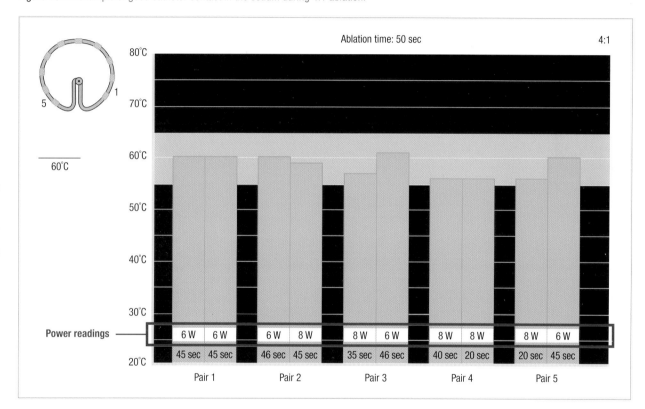

Low power delivery

In contrast, **Figure 14** shows an example on the generator screen of where high contact pressure on the PVAC array has pushed the electrode deep into the tissue and diminished the cooling effect of circulatory blood flow. Although the columns are all green, the delivered power is <4 W. RF energy delivery should be interrupted for safety and efficacy reasons and the catheter repositioned (eg, withdrawn slightly).

Figure 14. An example of low power delivery is likely because of poor electrode cooling from circulatory blood as a result of high contact force.

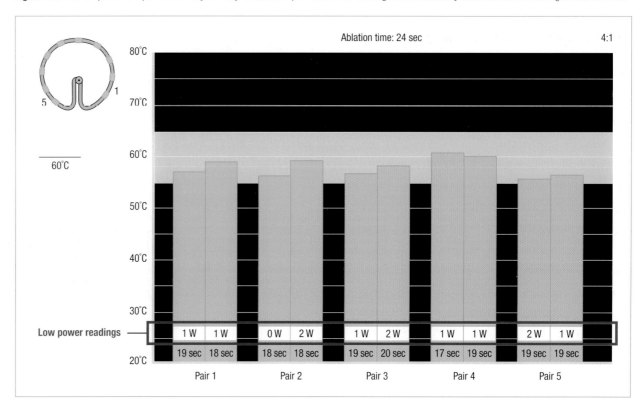

Low temperature readings

Figure 15 shows an example on the generator screen of a low temperature (blue color) for all of the columns despite delivery of good energy values. In this case, a decision needs to be made as to whether to continue the application or to stop and reposition the catheter. It is recommended that: (i) the application be stopped if the temperature is <50°C because the electrodes are most likely to be in contact with the blood pool, and (ii) to continue the application if the temperature is between 50°C and 55°C because the catheter electrodes are most likely to have good contact with the ostium in an area of high blood flow. Of course, local electrogram morphology and amplitude before ablation should also be taken into consideration when making a decision.

Figure 15. An example of a low temperature for all electrodes despite delivery of good energy values.

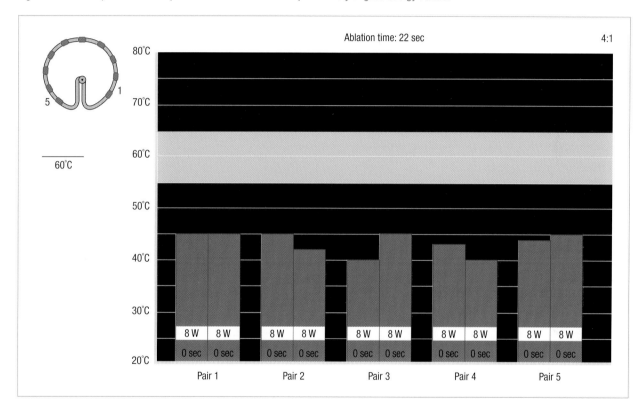

Low power on some electrode pairs

Figure 16 shows an example on the generator screen where all of the columns are green but some indicate very low power (ie, pairs 1 and 5). These electrodes are likely to be embedded too deeply in the tissue, and the respective electrode pairs should be deselected during ablation because this application will not produce a sufficient lesion size at that site.

Consistently low power at the same electrode, even after catheter movement, should raise the suspicion that char may have formed on that electrode. In such a situation the catheter should be withdrawn and carefully inspected. Also, large discrepancies in power output between neighboring electrodes (eg, 1 W/8 W at adjacent electrodes) may indicate char formation. In such a case, the catheter should be inspected before additional lesions are made.

Figure 16. An example showing very low power for electrode pairs 1 and 5.

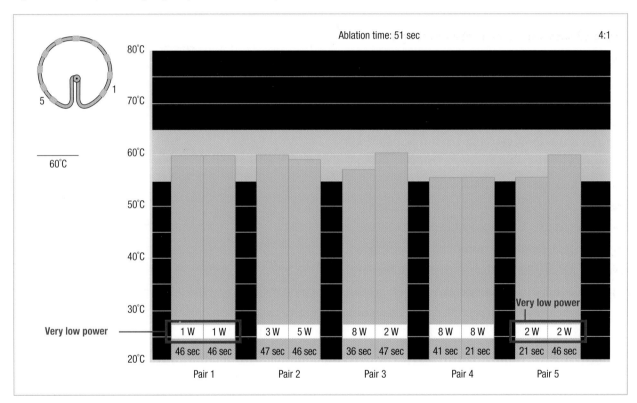

Temporary vein isolation

Figure 17 shows an example of an electrogram that could be expected after an inadequate lesion has been produced—at termination of the energy application, the PV potential has temporarily disappeared. However, after a few seconds, the potential reappears in the last two beats (with some delay in respect to the far-field atrial potential). In this kind of situation, optimizing catheter contact and repeating the energy application (including not only for the electrode pairs that showed the earliest potential [pairs 4 and 5] but also for the neighboring electrode pairs) will achieve a permanent isolation of the vein. One alternative option would be to use an RF energy delivery ratio of 2:1.

Figure 17. An electrogram showing production of an inadequate lesion following application. The PV potentials reappear (↓) (with some delay).

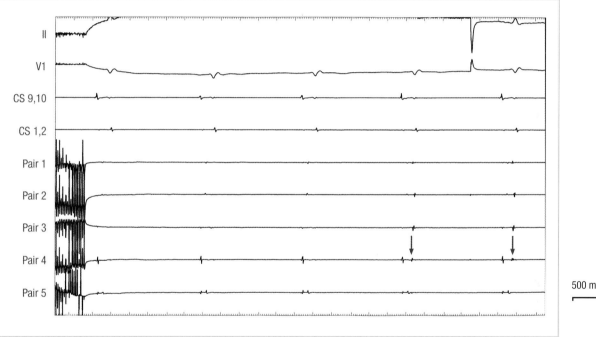

500 msec

Conclusion

- Several small independent electrodes in an array form a "virtual electrode" which allows long lesions to be safely created

- Current density for small electrodes with low power (~10 W) is comparable with larger electrodes

- Duty cycling allows electrode cooling and power modulation

- Phasing allows for simultaneous unipolar and bipolar energy application modes

- Fields allow mixing of unipolar and bipolar energy application modes to achieve different pre-defined energy ratios

- Lesion depth/fill can be controlled by using the appropriate energy mode

2 | Fluoroscopic Anatomy of the Left Atrium

This chapter describes the anatomy of the left atrium, as observed by the operator using fluoroscopy during an electrophysiological procedure. The topics included in this chapter should facilitate the operator in carrying out the procedure and improving safety.

Learning Objectives

> *To understand the orientation of the heart and the left atrium in the thorax*

> *To appreciate the angulation of the pulmonary vein ostia*

> *To be able to extrapolate the three-dimensional anatomy of the left atrium from two-dimensional fluoroscopic projections*

Introduction

When performing atrial fibrillation (AF) ablation using the Pulmonary Vein Ablation Catheter (PVAC), a precise appreciation of the anatomy of the left atrium (LA) and the pulmonary veins (PVs) is necessary because in most cases the procedure is performed without a three-dimensional navigation system. Therefore, the ability to extrapolate the three-dimensional LA anatomy from two-dimensional fluoroscopic projections is essential.

This chapter illustrates the basic anatomy in respect to PV isolation techniques when using either a conventional catheter or the PVAC. An understanding of the fundamental principles of the LA anatomy facilitates the handling of the catheter and avoids complications such as perforation of the LA roof. Proper use of direct maneuvers that target the PV ostium at the correct angle and orientation will reduce the amount of time required for fluoroscopy and for the procedure itself.

Throughout the chapter fluorograms of the LA are shown in both left anterior oblique (LAO) 45° and right anterior oblique (RAO) 30° projections without cranial or caudal angulation (*see* Tang et al 2010 in *Recommended Reading*).

The LAO projection is the view more appropriate for differentiating between the right atrium and the LA because the inter-atrial septum is projected between them (**Figure 1a**). In this view, the full length of the coronary sinus (CS) is observed as curving around the mitral valve; the tricuspid valve is seen as a full circle. On viewing from the top to the bottom in this plane, the ventricles appear to be in front of the atria and both overlap.

The RAO projection is optimal for differentiating the atria from the ventricles and shows the CS lying in the atrioventricular groove between them (**Figure 1b**). It is often viewed in a short projection.

Figure 1. Projections of the heart in (a) LAO and (b) RAO views.

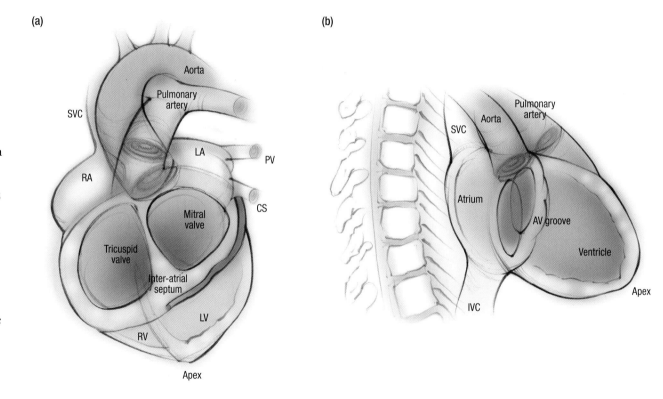

AV: atrioventricular; IVC: inferior vena cava; LV: left ventricle; RA: right atrium; RV: right ventricle; SVC: superior vena cava.

How to Produce a Pulmonary Vein Angiogram

In order to visualize all four PVs *simultaneously*, contrast agent is injected into the LA during asystole following administration of 12–18 mg of adenosine, or during rapid ventricular pacing. Care must be taken to ensure that the transseptal sheath is rotated posteriorly towards the smooth part of the LA so that the contrast agent can diffuse towards the PVs and not move anteriorly towards the mitral valve. Where diffusion of the contrast agent is incomplete, then subtle rotations of the sheath can facilitate filling of the agent into the PVs.

When carrying out *selective* PV angiograms, all four PVs can be injected separately with the aid of a steerable sheath. If a nonsteerable sheath is used, the upper PVs can easily be injected, whereas the lower PVs can be visualized at the ostium by carrying out a subtle posterior rotation of the sheath and pulling it back inferiorly. Alternatively, a flexible, multipurpose catheter may be advanced over a guidewire. However, the fastest way to identify all veins simultaneously is by injection of contrast agent into the LA during asystole.

Figure 2a shows an example of a PV angiogram with simultaneous visualization of all veins and the LA during asystole (following adenosine injection). Filling of the LA and PVs with contrast agent is optimal because the agent is not washed out. The PVAC sits in the superior vena cava and a temperature probe is located in the esophagus to illustrate the proximity of these structures. **Figure 2b** shows angiogram images of the PVs during rapid ventricular pacing, taken in both LAO and RAO projections.

Figure 2. Angiograms of **(a)** the LA and PVs, and **(b)** the PVs in asystole in **(i)** LAO and **(ii)** RAO views.

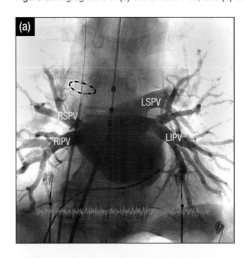

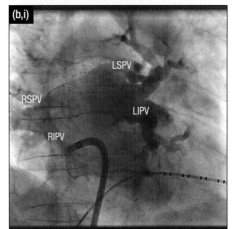
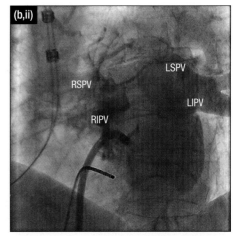

LIPV: left inferior pulmonary vein; LSPV: left superior pulmonary vein; RIPV: right inferior pulmonary vein; RSPV: right superior pulmonary vein.

Position of the Left Atrium and the Pulmonary Veins in the Frontal Plane

In the frontal view the LA has an oblique roof, which means that the position of the right superior pulmonary vein (RSPV) is lower than that of the left superior pulmonary vein (LSPV). Perforation at the atrial roof near to the RSPV can occur if the operator assumes that the roof is horizontal (**Figure 3**).

Angulation of the heart to the left side of the patient, which leads to an oblique roof, appears to be more prevalent in elderly patients because of a shortened vertebral column. As the thoracic cavity becomes shorter the heart rotates more

to the left side of the body. This may pose problems for the operator when making the transseptal puncture because the fossa ovalis is rotated more posteriorly.

Figure 3. (b) The atrial roof axis *in situ* where the RSPV is lower than the LSPV.

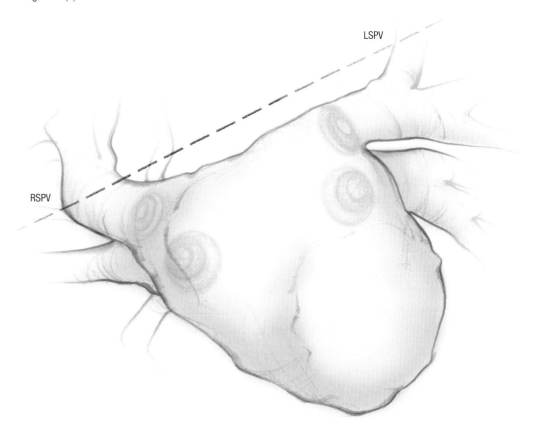

Figure 3. (a) Angiogram showing the position of the LA and PVs in the RAO view. With the vertebral column having been shortened because of scoliosis and osteoporosis, a possible increase in the rotation of the heart to the left side of the patient may result.

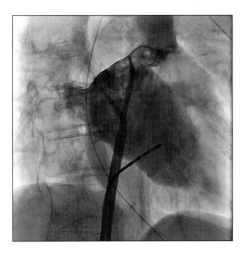

Orientation of the Heart in the Transversal Plane

The rotation of the heart in the transversal plane turns the right atrium and the right ventricle anteriorly, and consequently the LA and left ventricle are located posteriorly (**Figure 4**). Again, this rotation of the heart may seem to be more prevalent in elderly patients with osteoporosis and a short thorax. Therefore, the ostia of right-sided PVs might be positioned anteriorly to the ostia of the left-sided PVs. This means that in order to move the catheter from the left-sided PVs to the right-sided PVs, a clockwise rotation should be accompanied by a gradual withdrawal because the right-sided PVs are closer to the transseptal site.

Figure 4. A computed tomography (CT) scan showing the orientation of the heart in the transversal plane.

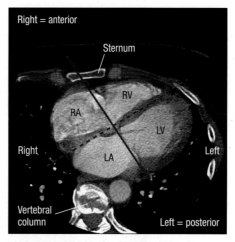

LV: left ventricle; RA: right atrium; RV: right ventricle.
Provided courtesy of Dr Manfred Rütschle, Clinic Im Park, Zurich, Switzerland.

The relative rotation and angulation of the heart is variable

Oblique orientation of the heart in the frontal and transversal planes is relative and depends on the size of the heart and the rotation to the left. Therefore, in those individuals who have small heart dimensions and a long thorax (ie, young people), the orientation of the heart is almost at the midline and the roof of the LA is more horizontal.

Figure 5 shows an example of a young patient with the heart having a relatively small angulation, a less oblique atrial roof, and a position close to the midline in the transversal plane.

Figure 5. Relative rotation and angulation of the heart is variable. **(a)** A CT view in the frontal plane of the LA and upper PVs. Note that in this young patient the atrial roof is less oblique than that for the patient depicted in Figure 3. **(b)** A CT scan showing a transverse view of the thorax as seen from beneath. Note that the angulation to the left side of the patient is minimal.

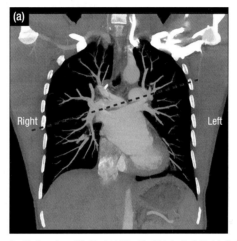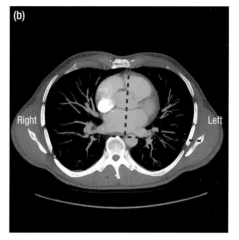

Provided courtesy of Dr Manfred Rütschle, Clinic Im Park, Zurich, Switzerland.

Positional Level of the Ostia of the Pulmonary Veins

The positions of the ostia of the upper PVs (LSPV and RSPV) are more lateral than those of the left inferior pulmonary vein (LIPV) and right inferior pulmonary vein (RIPV). This is because the inferior PVs point posteriorly directly into the lungs. Anterior to the left-sided PVs is the left atrial appendage (LAA). Between the left-sided PVs and the LAA is the LAA ridge, which can have a steep gradient that makes it difficult to obtain a steady catheter position (**Figure 6**). In this scenario, using the PVAC has the advantage that the guidewire can stabilize the catheter in the PV ostium thereby preventing it from being dislodged into the LAA.

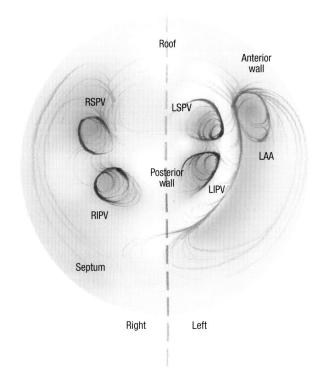

Figure 6. The inferior PVs are closer to the midline than the superior PVs.

Gross Concept of Left Atrial Anatomy in the Frontal Plane

In essence, the anatomy of the LA and the PVs is such that:

- The left atrial roof is oblique so that right-sided PVs are caudal to left-sided PVs in the frontal plane (**Figure 7a**)

- The lower PVs are posterior and positioned towards the midline versus the superior PVs, which are positioned anterior and more laterally. This is in contrast to the horizontal view of the LA often presented in three-dimensional geometrical maps where the ostia of the PVs are shown as being at the same level (**Figure 7b**)

Figure 7. (a) Left atrial anatomy in the anteroposterior view; note the orientation in the body. (b) Posterior aspect of the virtual LA geometry by a three-dimensional mapping system.

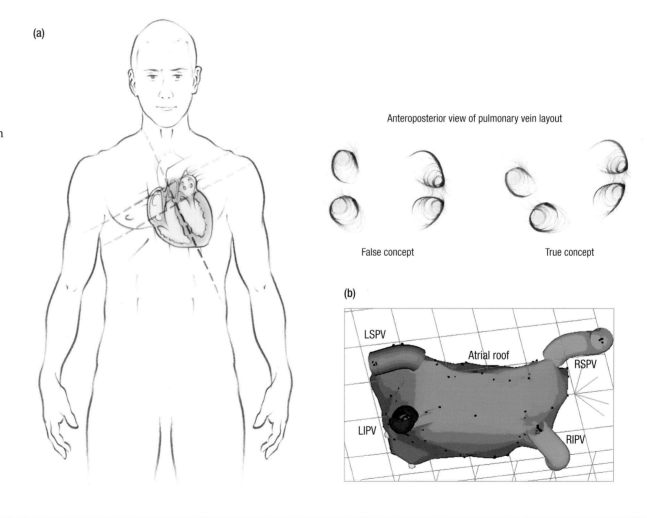

(a)

Anteroposterior view of pulmonary vein layout

False concept

True concept

(b)

LSPV

Atrial roof

RSPV

LIPV

RIPV

The Location of the Lung Lobes Determines the Orientation of Corresponding Pulmonary Veins

The distribution of the lung lobes determines the location of the PVs draining from the corresponding lobe (**Figure 8**). The superior lobes are located anteriorly; the inferior lobes are located posteriorly. The right middle lobe is located anteriorly, draining in 15–30% of individuals via a separate right middle PV (RMPV). The lateral views show the inferior lobes (blue) and superior lobes (green), with the corresponding veins in the same color. The ostia of the superior PVs and the inferior PVs may be positioned at the same level in the craniocaudal direction, but angulated anteriorly (superior PVs) and posteriorly (inferior PVs). Therefore, it may be more appropriate to rename the PVs as *anterior PVs* instead of superior PVs and *posterior PVs* instead of inferior PVs (**Figures 8** and **9**).

Figure 8. Location of the lung lobes and PVs in the lateral view.

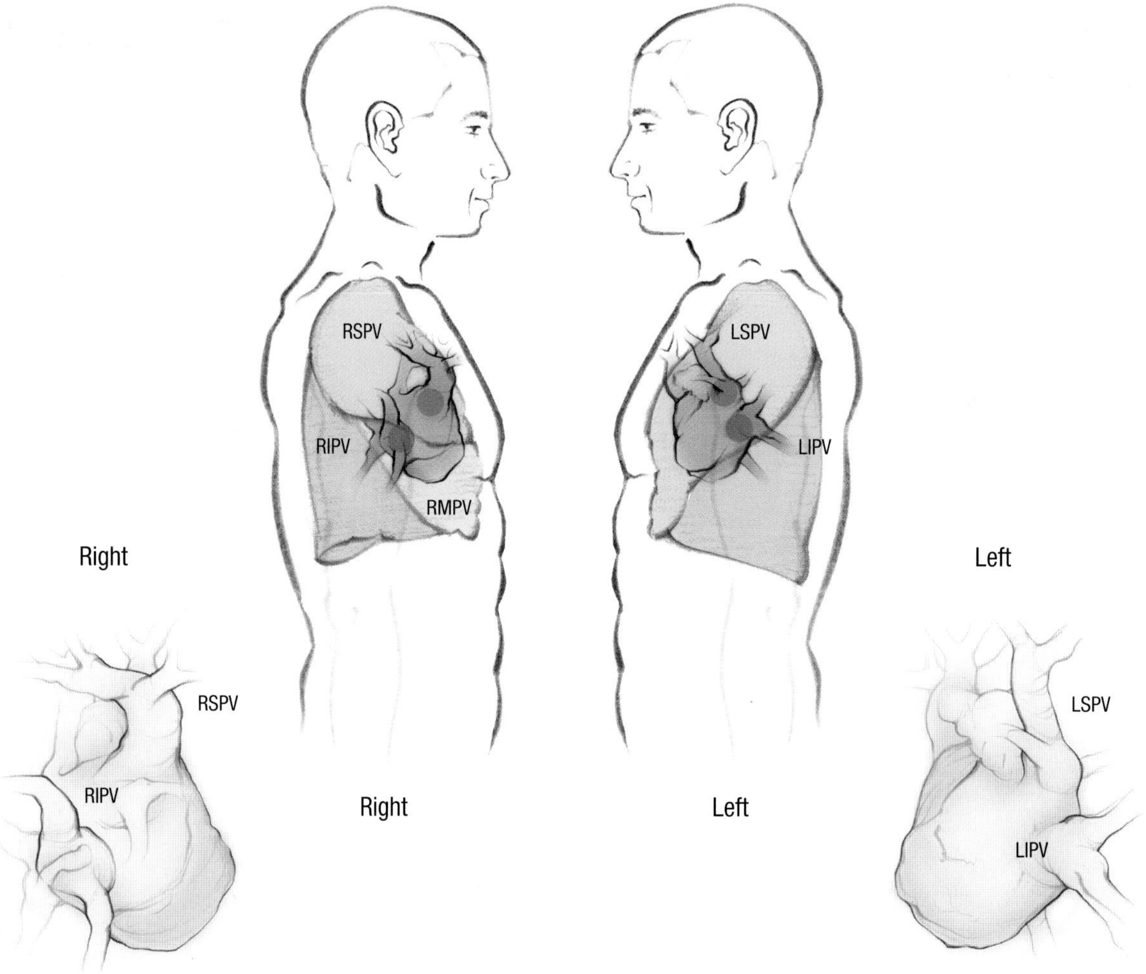

Figure 9 shows that in the RAO projection, the ostium of the LSPV is positioned at nearly the same level as that of the LIPV. However, the ostium of the LSPV is directed anteriorly towards the observer in the LAO projection, while the LIPV is directed posteriorly. In this patient, the separation of the two ostia appears to be more distinct in the LAO projection. As it is difficult to appreciate the angulated "take-off" of PV ostia using two-dimensional fluoroscopy, it may become necessary to view the projections at different angles.

Figure 9. The ostia of the LSPV and the LIPV in (a) LAO and (b) RAO views. Note that there are two sheaths, one in each PV.

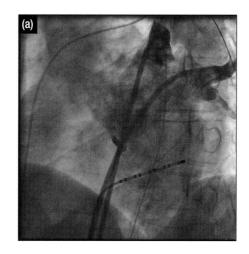
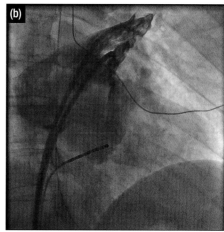

Differentiation of the Ostia of the Pulmonary Veins

On viewing the ostia of the PVs on opposite (LAO and RAO) fluoroscopic angulations, the orientation of both the inferior and superior PVs becomes clearer. The right-sided PVs can be differentiated by LAO views (**Figure 10a**). In LAO, the RSPV points anteriorly to the left side of the screen and the ostium is projected as a narrow oval. In contrast, the RIPV points away from the viewer towards the vertebral column. The result is that the RIPV ostium is projected as a full circle. Correspondingly, the left-sided PVs can be differentiated by RAO views (**Figure 10b**).

Figure 10. (a) The LAO view differentiates the right-sided PVs, and (b) the RAO view differentiates the left-sided PVs (the LSPV projects anteriorly to the right and the LIPV projects posteriorly).

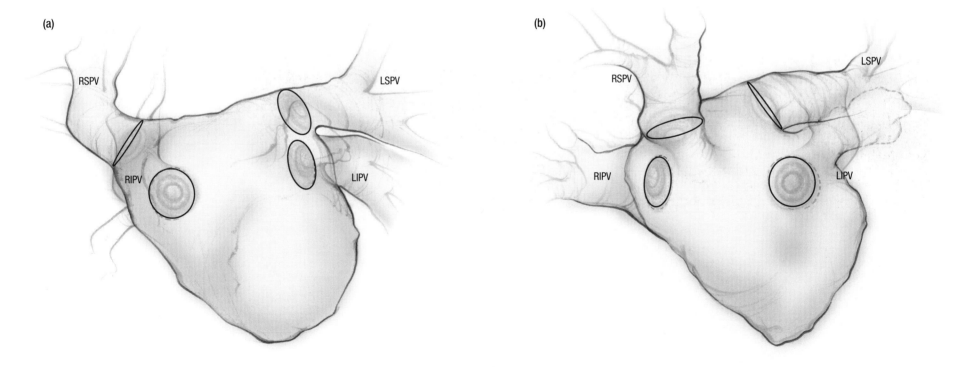

Figure 11 shows selective angiograms of the LSPV and LIPV in both LAO and RAO views. For the LSPV (**Figure 11a**), in the LAO projection, the ostium is orientated to the border of the cardiac shadow, which means that differentiation between the LSPV and LIPV cannot be easily made. The RAO projection is more useful and shows that the LSPV is taking off from the LA in the anterior direction, away from the vertebral column.

For LIPV (**Figure 11b**), in the LAO projection, the ostium of the LIPV is not orientated to the border of the cardiac shadow, but is located more inside the cardiac shadow because it is closer to the midline of the LA. Thus, the LIPV is most likely to receive radiofrequency (RF) energy ablation inside the vein and is, therefore, highly prone to stenosis on using conventional RF ablation. The differentiation between LSPV and LIPV is more distinct in the RAO projection, with the LIPV being orientated away from the viewer (posterior angulation), resulting in a circular ostium projection.

Figure 11. Fluoroscopic scans showing (a) the LSPV, and (b) the LIPV in (i) LAO and (ii) RAO views. The projections of the ostia are shown as oval or circular.

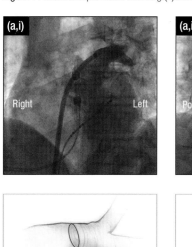
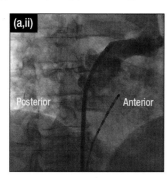
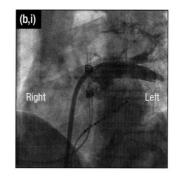
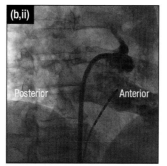
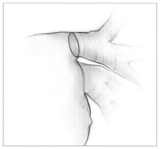
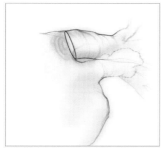
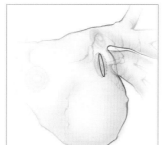
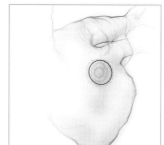

Figure 12 shows selective angiograms of the RSPV and RIPV in both LAO and RAO views. In **Figure 12a**, the ostium of the RSPV is projected to the border of the cardiac shadow in the RAO view. The RAO projection can make it difficult to discern from the RIPV if the latter is taking off at a similar level and has a large superior branch. The LAO view is more useful because the orientation of the RSPV points anteriorly away from the vertebral column, which is in contrast to that of the RIPV, which points posteriorly.

In **Figure 12b**, in the LAO view the posterior take-off of the RIPV means that the ostium is observed as a full circle, which goes directly into the plane. As with the LIPV, the ostium of the RIPV in LAO and RAO views is projected not at the border of the cardiac shadow, but rather is located a little more inside. This means that it would be easy to inadvertently advance the catheter too far into the vein.

Figure 12. Fluoroscopic scans showing (a) the RSPV, and (b) the RIPV in (i) LAO and (ii) RAO views. The projections of the ostia are shown as oval or circular.

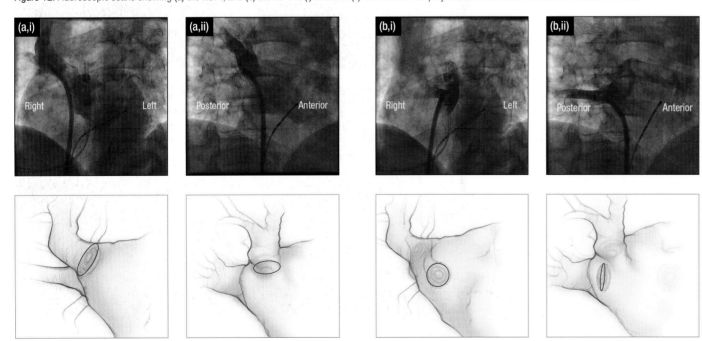

Distinguishing between the left atrial appendage and the left superior pulmonary vein

It is possible that a single plane misjudgment could occur where the LAA is mistaken for a PV. **Figure 13** shows how the LAA and the LSPV can sometimes be mixed up, particularly when they appear superimposed in the LAO projection. This mistake can lead to a risk of perforation of the thin wall of the LAA.

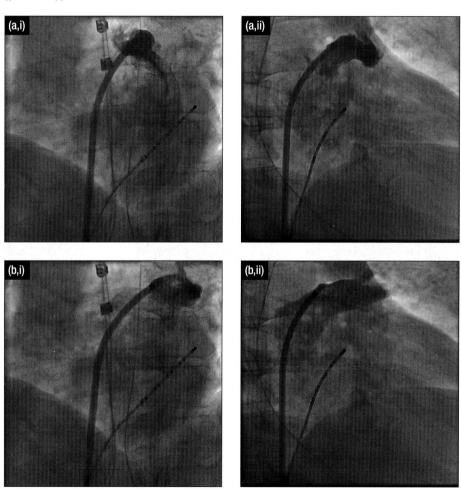

Figure 13. (a) The LAA and (b) the LSPV can sometimes be mixed up even when viewed in two projections. (i) LAO and (ii) RAO views.

In order to prevent such a mishap the "guidewire test" is recommended before advancing any catheter or sheath (**Figure 14**). If the guidewire goes beyond the border of the cardiac shadow its position lies inside the PV. If the guidewire stays within the cardiac shadow then it may well be situated inside the LAA, in which case the guidewire should be withdrawn and readvanced in another direction. The use of the guidewire test during mapping with the PVAC offers a unique advantage over conventional circular mapping catheters.

Figure 14. The guidewire test can help to distinguish between **(a)** the LAA (RAO view), and **(b)** the LSPV (LAO view).

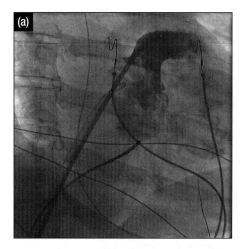
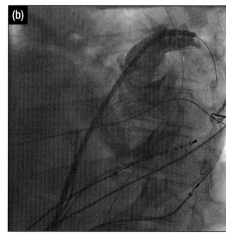

The Pulmonary Veins and the Esophagus

The proximity of the esophagus to the LA has important implications for RF energy delivery (**Figure 15**). Because of their anatomical relationship, which can be very close, the RF energy delivery should be limited to a 4:1 ratio whenever ablating near the posterior wall of the LA. The esophagus has a variable course, and can, therefore, move during the procedure from a position close to the right-sided PVs to one close to the left-sided PVs, and back again.

Figure 16 shows an example where the esophagus is within 3 mm of the LIPV, which is one electrode length of the PVAC. The spatial position of the esophagus can be observed by the location of a nasogastric tube (←).

The PVAC is located in the LIPV. In this case, both LAO and RAO views show that the nasogastric tube lies within a few millimeters of the PVAC. For this reason it is recommended that only a 4:1 RF energy ratio is employed at this location because ablation in this area may carry a higher risk profile with a greater chance for collateral damage when using an energy mode with a greater unipolar ratio.

Figure 15. The esophagus is highlighted with barium contrast agent and is located behind the RSPV in which the PVAC is situated. (a) LAO and (b) RAO views.

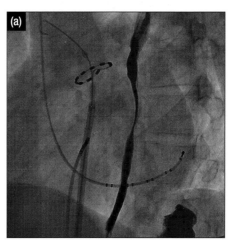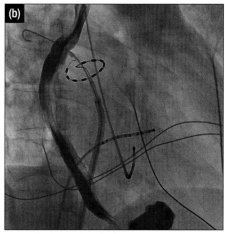

Figure 16. Close proximity of the esophagus and the LIPV. (a) LAO and (b) RAO views.

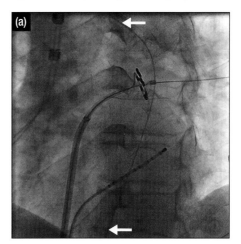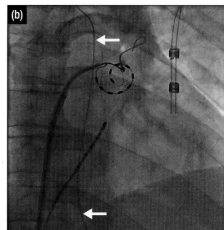

The Ostium and Antrum of the Pulmonary Vein

The ostium of a PV is defined as the intersection of the tangents from the PVs and the LA (**Figure 17a**). Proximal to that line is the antrum and distal to the line is the PV trunk.

Figure 17b shows the PV ostium (blue oval) and antrum (red oval). Note that the PVs form a continuum with the smooth part of the LA, both histologically and macroscopically. As a consequence, the functional properties of the antrum and PV may be similar, and therefore, firing foci can also be found in the antra of PVs.

In addition, muscle fibers are routed directly from the antrum to the PV. Thus, effective isolation of the PV can be achieved by interrupting those muscle fibers at the antral level. This is indicative of the anatomy of the antrum having equal importance to that of the PV.

Figure 17c is a post-mortem anatomical preparation showing the continuum of the antrum and the PV, which is the site for ablation with RF energy using both conventional catheters and the PVAC.

Figure 17. (a) A three-dimensional CT model of the LA and the PV (*see* Scharf et al 2003 in *Recommended Reading*). The ostium of a PV is defined as the intersection of the tangents from the PVs (green) and the LA (red). (b) A catheter can be placed in the antrum for ablation (red oval) and in the PV ostium for mapping (blue oval). (c) A post-mortem anatomical preparation showing a continuum formed between the antrum and the PVs.

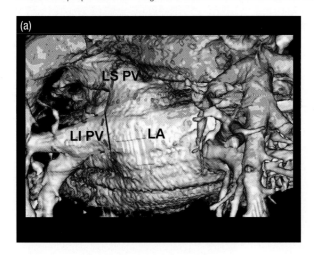
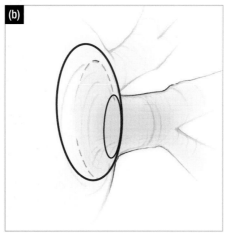
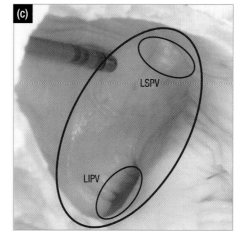

Provided courtesy of Dr Maxim Viktorovitch Didenko, St Petersburg, Russia.

The Common Ostium

As a consequence of the left-sided PVs bridging over the descending aorta, these PVs split more distally into branches than do the right-sided PVs (**Figure 18a**). This may be the reason that a common ostium occurs more frequently on the left side. The common ostium is defined by a large trunk and a split into the LSPV and LIPV occurring not at the atrial level (↓¹) but approximately 1 cm distally (↓²) towards the lungs.

In cases where there is a common ostium the ablation is performed at the antral level, as indicated in **Figure 17**. Of note is the fact that the diameter of the common ostium is larger than the 25 mm diameter of the PVAC. This means that antral isolation requires active curving of the catheter and rotation around the entire circumference of the vein to achieve isolation (**Figure 19**).

Figure 18. (a) Venograms ([i] LAO and [ii] RAO views) showing the outlines of the ostia (represented by red ovals) and the LA wall (green curve), and (b) an anatomical preparation showing a common ostium.

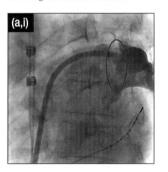 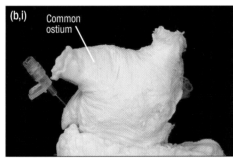
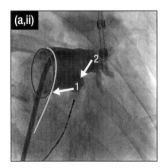 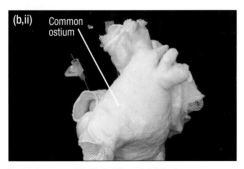

Provided courtesy of Dr Maxim Viktorovitch Didenko, St Petersburg, Russia.

Figure 19. Ablation and mapping positions for the PVAC in the common left PV.

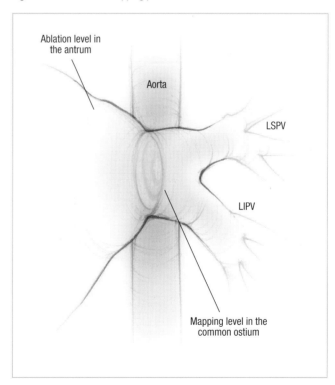

Conclusion

- The left atrial roof can be oblique, meaning that the right side is lower than the left side

- The superior PVs have a take-off in the anterior direction; the inferior PVs have a take-off in the posterior direction

- The ostia of the inferior PVs are located more towards the midline

- The esophagus can be very close to the left- or right-sided PVs and the posterior LA

3 | PVAC Management in Practice

This chapter provides a practical approach to the use of the Pulmonary Vein Ablation Catheter (PVAC), sheath, and guidewire to facilitate the creation of an optimal set of ablation lesions.

Learning Objectives

> *To comprehend the specifications and utilization of the PVAC in practice following explanation of the ablation procedure*

> *To understand the essential equipment for catheter ablation in practice together with the basic options*

> *To appreciate the manipulation of the catheter for specific pulmonary veins in specific anatomical situations*

> *To understand the handling options of the catheter system and how this will facilitate pulmonary vein isolation by ablation in the antrum*

The PVAC

The PVAC has the following technical specifications:

- A 9 F catheter shaft, with a length of 160 cm (**Figure 1**)

- A hollow shaft for over-the-wire handling

- A guidewire introduction via the back end (**Figure 2a**)

- A connector at the back end to attach to the catheter cable (**Figure 2a**)

- Bidirectional steering through use of the steering knob on the left-hand side of the catheter grip (**Figure 2b**)

  - Pushing the steering knob forwards turns the shaft down; pulling it backwards turns the shaft up (**Figure 2c**)

- The tip can be extended by the slide control knob on the top surface of the catheter grip (**Figure 2d**)

  - Moving the slide control knob forward extends the tip until it becomes helical

- A 10 electrode spiral array with a diameter of 25 mm (**Figure 2e**)

- Platinum electrodes, length 3 mm, diameter 1.5 mm, spacing 3 mm (**Figure 2e**)

- A thermocouple at the anterior surface of each electrode

- A capture device to facilitate the introduction of the extended array into the sheath (**Figures 2f** and **5a**)

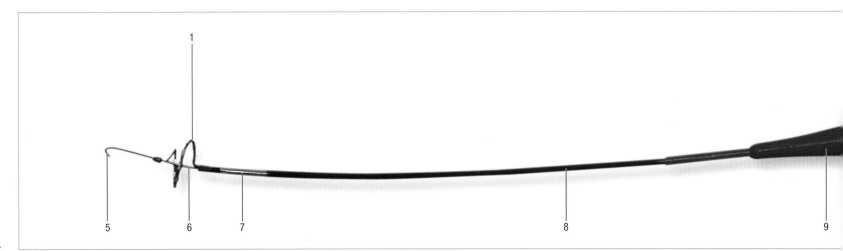

Figure 1. The complete PVAC device.

Components of the PVAC device

1. 10-Electrode array
2. Steering knob
3. Slide control knob
4. Connector
5. Guidewire
6. Inner shaft of guidewire lumen
7. Braided section
8. 9 F shaft
9. Capture device
10. Shaft
11. Ergonomic hand grip
12. Guidewire luer hub

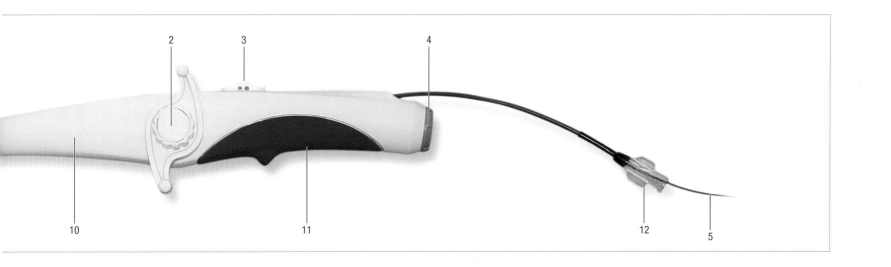

Figure 2. Specific attributes of the PVAC. **(a)** Guidewire introduction, **(b)** steering knob, **(c)** steering knob options, **(d)** slide control knob, **(e)** 10 electrode spiral array with electrode pairing and dimensions shown, and **(f)** tip extended from the sheath.

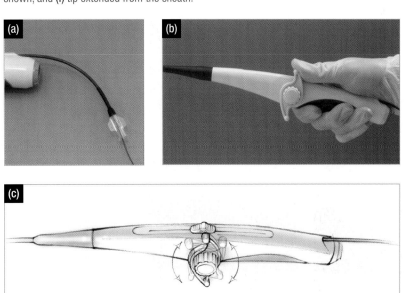

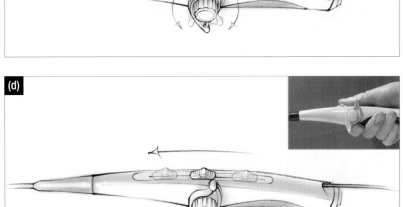

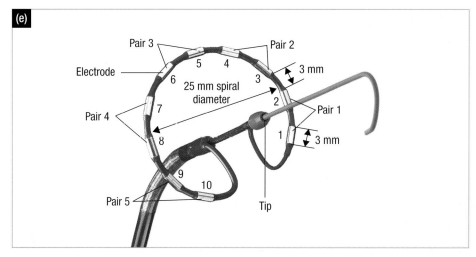

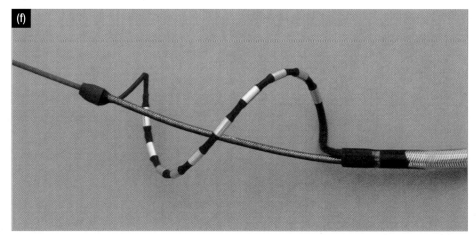

Transsseptal Sheath and Guidewire

The sheath and guidewire for the PVAC have the following technical specifications:

- Any sheath should have an inner lumen diameter of at least 9.5 F, side-holes, and a working length of >60 cm compatible with the PVAC

- The sheath has a braided body for improved torque and catheter support

- A double valve to prevent retrograde leaking

- A side opening to flush out the sheath

- Steerable sheath:

  - Use steerability of either the steerable sheath, PVAC shaft, or both (the PVAC should never be steered in the sheath)

  - Selective cannulation of individual pulmonary veins (PVs) (**Figure 3**)

  - Flexibility for improved manipulation; free rotation of the PVAC itself

  - Potential to extend the sheath all the way up to the tip for better control and increased support

- Nonsteerable sheath:

  - Use steerability of the PVAC

  - Pull back the sheath to the septum/right atrium so that the steering part of the PVAC is free outside the sheath

- To facilitate smooth manipulation, a guidewire of preferably 0.032 inches diameter and at least 180 cm length should be used

- A guidewire is used for selective cannulation in PV side branches and for stabilizing the PVAC in the antrum

Figure 3. Selective cannulation of individual PVs (left anterior oblique [LAO] and right anterior oblique [RAO] views).

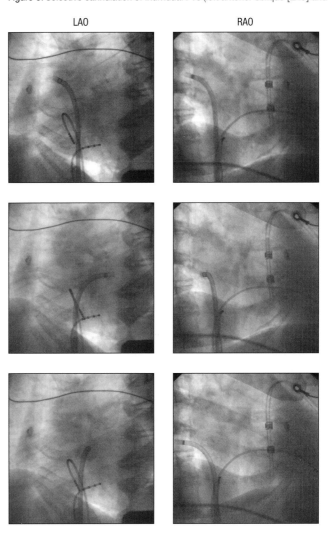

LAO   RAO

Deployment of the PVAC in the Left Atrium

Making the transseptal puncture:

- Introduce a multipolar catheter inside the coronary sinus (CS) to delineate the mitral annulus

- Introduce the guidewire transfemorally into the superior vena cava (SVC)

- Exchange the introducer with the transseptal sheath

- Introduce the sheath over the wire into the SVC (**Figure 4a**)

- Introduce a transseptal needle inside the sheath (**Figure 4b**)

- Gradually pull back the sheath until the tip falls into the fossa ovalis (**Figure 4c**)

- Pull back the tip of the sheath to a low septal position posterior to above the CS ostium

- Aim the transseptal puncture posterior and parallel to the CS (**Figure 4d**)

- Extend the sheath over the needle across the septum into the left atrium (LA) (**Figure 4e**)

- Pull back the introducer (**Figure 4f**) and inject contrast agent to ascertain the LA position ensuring that the sheath is inside the LA and that there is no pericardial effusion (**Figure 4g**)

Figure 4. Making the transseptal passage.

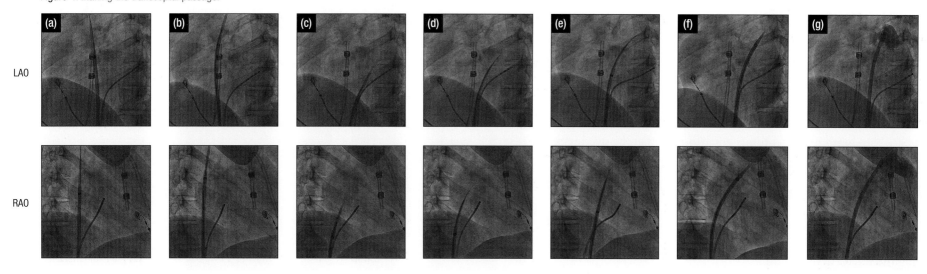

Using the PVAC:

- As the capture device is advanced forward, continue to progress the slide control knob forward to extend the spiral array. Make sure that it is extended completely to avoid fracture of the distal wire (**Figure 5a**)

- Introduce the capture device into the sheath and advance the catheter towards the LA

- Introduce the guidewire into the left superior pulmonary vein (LSPV) (**Figure 5b**) and advance the PVAC from the sheath while retracting the slide control knob (**Figure 5c,d**). The spiral array will deploy into the antrum (**Figure 5e**)

- The guidewire should always be extended from the PVAC tip to prevent curving and distortion of the spiral array (**Figure 5f**)

- Remove the capture device from the sheath and replace it on the catheter handle

Figure 5. (a) If the capture device extends over the tip then this can lead to a potential fracture of the distal wire. (b–e) Advancing the guidewire into the LSPV and deploying the catheter tip into the antrum, and (f) inappropriate extension of the PVAC without first extending the guidewire.

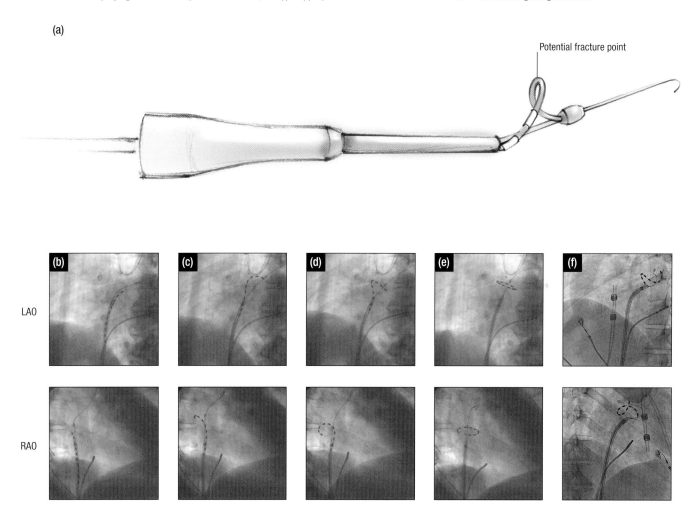

Shape and Steerability of the PVAC

- The PVAC shaft has bidirectional steerability (180° curve) achieved by using the steering knob (*see* **Figure 2b**)

- The slide control knob on the top surface of the catheter handle extends the spiral array to make it more helical (*see* **Figure 2d**)

- Rotation of the catheter can change the diameter of the spiral array, making it smaller (clockwise) or larger (counter-clockwise) (**Figure 6a**)

- When the electrodes overlap (**Figure 6b**), one of the pairs should be deselected during ablation to prevent radiofrequency (RF) energy from causing a short circuit between the electrodes

- By extending the tip into the PV, the proximal electrodes may improve contact during ablation. The electrodes inside the vein should be deselected during ablation (**Figure 6c**)

- Deflecting the PVAC shaft or the transseptal sheath will move the catheter array to the inferior end of the PV, while straightening the PVAC shaft or transseptal sheath will move the array to the superior end. Clockwise turning of the sheath will move the PVAC posteriorly for left-sided PVs and anteriorly for right-sided PVs, while counter-clockwise turning of the sheath will do the opposite (**Figure 6d**)

- When the PVAC shaft/sheath is curved it will make wider sweeps when rotated. This may facilitate ablation in the antrum, away from the ostium. For a common ostium, the spiral array can be used to cover the complete ostial region of the vein (**Figure 6e**). The guidewire may be positioned in the upper and lower branches of the vein

Figure 6. (a) Rotation of the PVAC can change the diameter of the catheter ring to enable it to adapt to the local anatomy, or extend deeper into the vein.

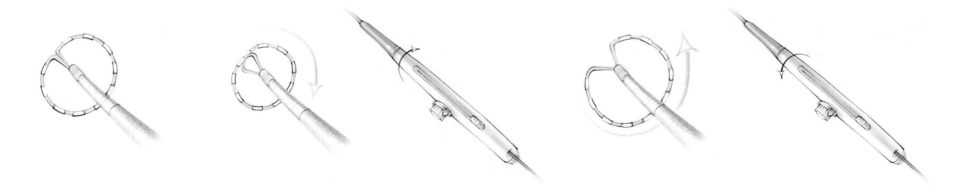

Figure 6. **(b)** Ablation should not be conducted on overlapping electrode pairs. **(c)** By extending the catheter tip into the PV, the proximal electrodes may improve contact during ablation. However, the electrode pairs positioned inside the vein must be deselected during ablation to avoid ablation inside the vein and the risk of PV stenosis. **(d)** Movement options for the PVAC in a left-sided vein, and **(e)** the catheter tip can be used to cover the complete ostial region of a vein even if it has a large diameter.

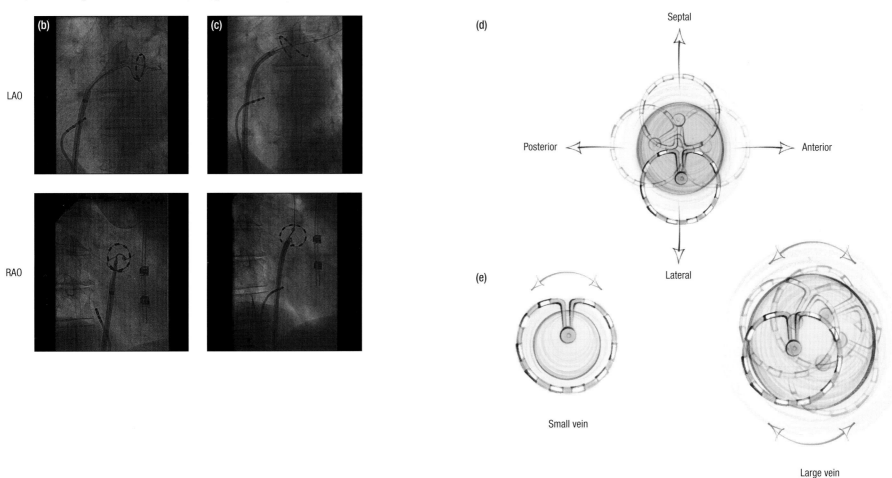

Ablation Using the PVAC

- Position the PVAC in such a way that all of the electrode pairs show local potentials. This will allow for optimal use of the full potential of the multielectrode array. Performing only segmental applications will slow down the procedure and may increase the occurrence of gaps, creating an ineffective line of block

- The standard RF energy mode for the PVAC is a 4:1 bipolar to unipolar ratio. A 2:1 bipolar to unipolar ratio setting creates deeper lesions, and may be selected when local potentials do not disappear in spite of there being good contact between the catheter and ostium and a temperature of >50°C

- By performing multiple applications using the complete electrode array of the catheter, the circular lesions will overlap (**Figure 7a**). In a small vein, the catheter ring of the PVAC may have a diameter sufficient to cover the complete ostium (*see* **Figure 6e**); simple rotation without curving the shaft may be sufficient to isolate the vein

- At least two catheter applications should be performed per vein and the PVAC rotated through 180°. This should overcome the development of any gap in the lesion between electrodes 1 and 10 where no bipolar energy can flow

- The goal of ablation is to eliminate all potentials inside the antrum leading to PV isolation

- When there is only a segment of the ostium with potentials still registering then place the middle electrode pair on that segment. Select the adjacent electrode pairs on either side for ablation during the application to sandwich that segment and to ensure that the maximum bipolar energy flows to the target electrodes (**Figure 7b** and **c**)

- Use the mantra "work with the catheter to make it work" by turning the PVAC shaft or the transseptal sheath clockwise and counter-clockwise, changing the shaft curve, rotating it clockwise and counter-clockwise, and extending the catheter tip

- During an application, if the target temperature is not reached after 10–15 sec despite maximum power, apply a slightly increased forward pressure on the catheter to increase the electrode contact and achieve the desired temperature

Figure 7. (a) Multiple applications ensure that lesions overlap. (b) "Sandwich" the target segment with the middle part of the PVAC. (i) Angiograms of the right inferior pulmonary vein (RIPV), and (ii) the PVAC in the RIPV.

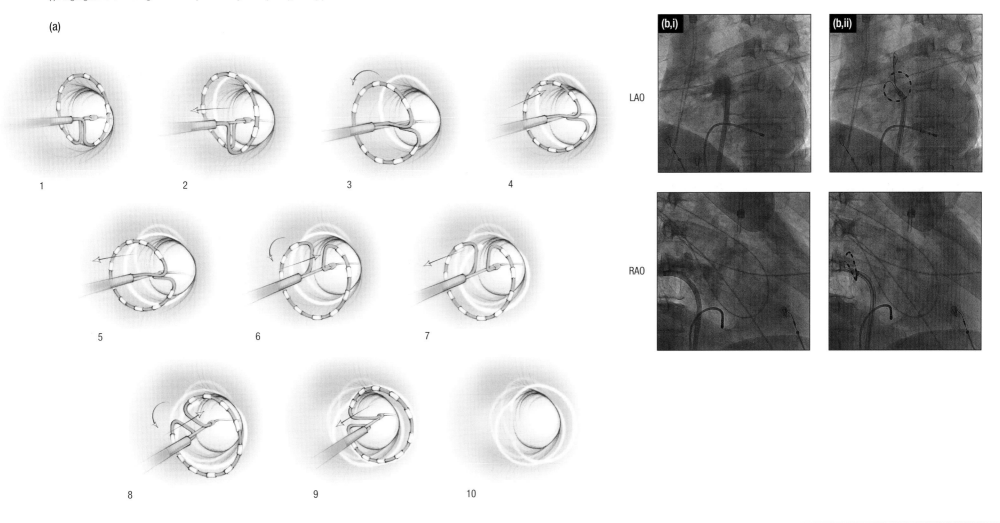

(a)

1 2 3 4

5 6 7

8 9 10

(b,i) (b,ii)

LAO

RAO

Figure 7. (c) "Sandwich" the target segment with the middle part of the PVAC. Tracings (i) before, and (ii) after ablation. Local PV potentials (∗), remote LA potentials (↓).

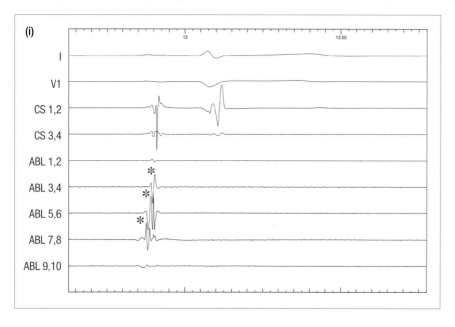

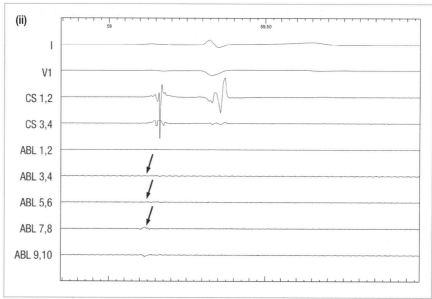

Targeting the Pulmonary Veins: General Concepts

- Use biplanar fluoroscopic images as a guide to stay outside the PV lumen

- The position of the PVAC in relation to the ostium of the PV can be determined based on (biplane) PV angiography. Alternatively, three-dimensional rotational angiography may provide a reliable anatomical image of the LA and the PVs to guide ablation (**Figure 8**)

- Push the PVAC into the antrum until resistance builds up and the catheter deforms or extends into the vein itself

- Extend the catheter (partially) inside the PV to establish the potentials prior to ablation (template mapping)

- Pull back the PVAC to establish where the catheter "pops" out of the vein and regains its original shape

- Feed the guidewire into different side branches of the PVs. This will allow a varied approach to the PV and extension into the antrum away from the ostium on all sides

- The antra of the PVs are usually close together and applications at the upper and lower antra will usually overlap. The more effort that is made for the upper vein, the less effort is usually needed to ablate the lower vein, and *vice versa*

- Several applications should be performed in both the upper and lower veins before moving to establish PV isolation because cross connections may remain that prevent selective isolation

Figure 8. Additional imaging modalities such as three-dimensional rotational angiography overlay may be used to verify the position of the PVAC relative to the ostium of the PV. (a) The PVAC in the LSPV and (b) in the right inferior pulmonary vein (RIPV).

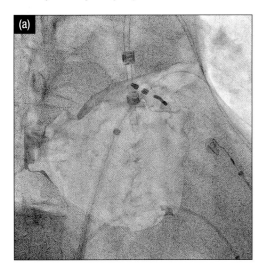
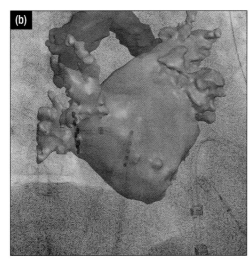

Targeting Pulmonary Veins: The Left Superior Pulmonary Vein

- Usually, the LSPV has a oblique/longitudinal upward "take-off" from the LA

- The guidewire is positioned in the upper side branch of the LSPV

- The spiral array of the PVAC is positioned parallel to the wall in both the LAO and RAO orientations (**Figure 9a**)

- With subsequent applications, the PVAC should target the tissue specifically at the lower and upper parts as well as the anterior and posterior parts of the vein antrum

- The carina between the LSPV and left inferior pulmonary vein (LIPV) is not targeted specifically, but will also be isolated as the lesions around the LSPV and LIPV eventually overlap. If there is no lesion on the carina, particularly if the carina is positioned outside the cardiac shadow, then an incomplete ablation lesion for either vein may lead to neither vein being isolated (**Figure 9b,i**)

- The ridge between the LSPV and the left atrial appendage (LAA) is not specifically targeted, but should be ablated as well. If the lesions do not encompass the ridge, a potential gap to the LAA may lead to failure of LSPV isolation (**Figure 9b,ii**)

- Caution should be taken when targeting PV potentials at the side of the LAA because remote signals could be misinterpreted as being local potentials. This could lead to an excessive number of applications and collateral damage

Figure 9. (a,i) An angiogram of the PV, (a,ii) the PVAC array is positioned parallel to the wall. (b) Incomplete ablation of either (i) the carina or (ii) the LAA ridge may lead to a failure to isolate the vein(s).

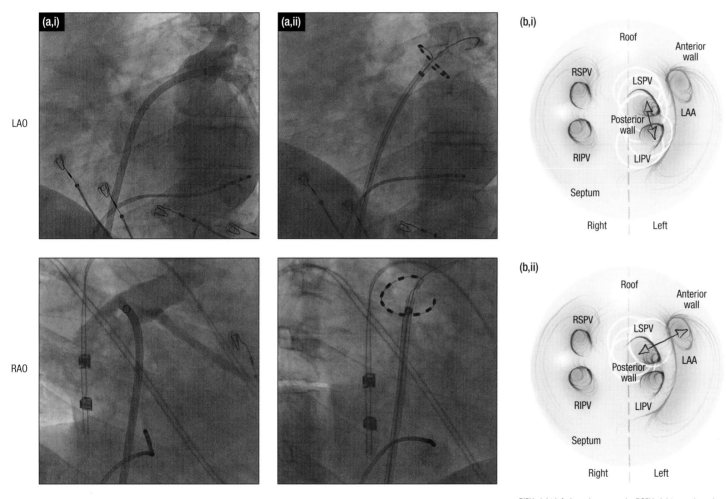

RIPV: right inferior pulmonary vein; RSPV: right superior pulmonary vein.

Targeting Pulmonary Veins: The Left Inferior Pulmonary Vein

- Usually, the LIPV has a steep perpendicular take-off from the wall of the LA

- Position the guidewire of the PVAC into the lower side branch of the LIPV (**Figure 10a,i** and **b**). During later applications a different approach to the vein can be achieved by positioning the guidewire in the upper side branch (**Figure 10a,ii**)

- When the electrodes of the catheter ring overlap then deselect one of the pairs

- Make a 90° angle with the shaft/sheath, and avoid approaching the PV from the superior side as this will hamper the ability to make contact with the vein antrum

- Position the PVAC perpendicular to the vein wall of the LIPV in the RAO orientation and anteroposterior in the LAO orientation

- Position the tip of the PVAC below the ostium during the first application(s). This will allow the catheter tip to extend and to touch the wall as the wall fades left to the annulus, thereby increasing contact (**Figure 10c**)

- If necessary, position the tip of the array inside the vein and rotate the PVAC counter-clockwise to enlarge the diameter of the spiral array and enable improved proximal contact (**Figure 10d**). In this way the lower and posterior parts of the antrum are targeted. Be sure to deselect any electrode pairs inside the vein during ablation

- **Figure 10b–d** shows that in the LAO orientation the PVAC remains proximal inside the cardiac shadow; otherwise, ablation would be performed distally inside the PV ostium

Figure 10. **(a)** Use of different side branches to obtain varied approaches to the PV.

(a,i)

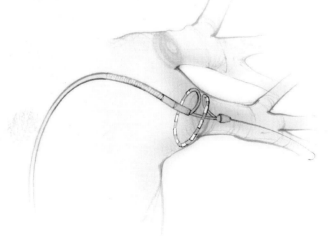

(a,ii)

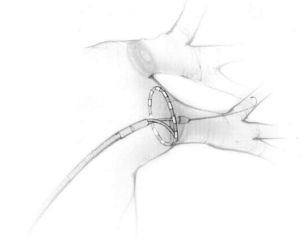

Figure 10. (b,i) An angiogram of the PV, (b,ii) positioning of the guidewire of the PVAC into the lower side branch of the LIPV. (c) In a separate patient the distal end of the PVAC array is extended below the ostium of the LIPV to ablate the lower rim, and (d) the catheter array may be positioned inside the vein to improve contact and ablation with the proximal pairs. Any pair inside the ostium is deselected for ablation. The panels (c,ii) show the PV angiograms for reference purposes for both (c) and (d).

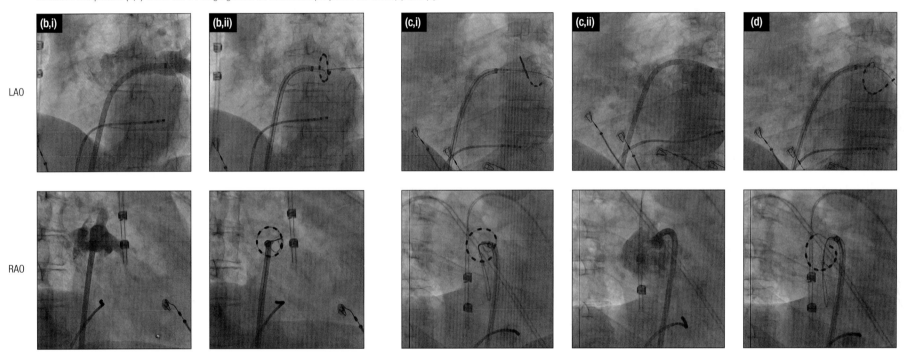

LAO

RAO

Targeting Pulmonary Veins: The Right Superior Pulmonary Vein

- Usually, the right superior pulmonary vein (RSPV) has an oblique take-off from the wall of the LA

- First, position the guidewire into the upper side branch of the RSPV (**Figure 11a**), then place it into other side branches during later applications

- Position the ring of the PVAC parallel to the wall of the RSPV in both LAO and RAO orientations (**Figure 11a**) in order to make the first circular applications

- Position the guidewire into the other side branches, and curve and/or rotate the catheter to make it larger and to cover the upper and lower part (**Figure 11b**) of the antrum of the RSPV

- By moving the sheath clockwise and counter-clockwise the septal and posterior parts of the antrum (**Figure 11b**) may be targeted (compare with **Figure 6d**)

- A separate vein, the right middle pulmonary vein (RMPV), may also be selectively targeted. It is usually located just below the RSPV projecting to the left in LAO and frontally in the RAO orientation (**Figure 11c**)

Figure 11. (a) The PVAC is positioned parallel to the wall of the RSPV to make initial applications, (b) enlarging the PVAC diameter and rotating the sheath to target all antral segments by opposing rotations. The panels (a,ii) show the PV angiograms for reference purposes for both (a) and (b). (c) Targeting the middle vein (RMPV) below the RSPV.

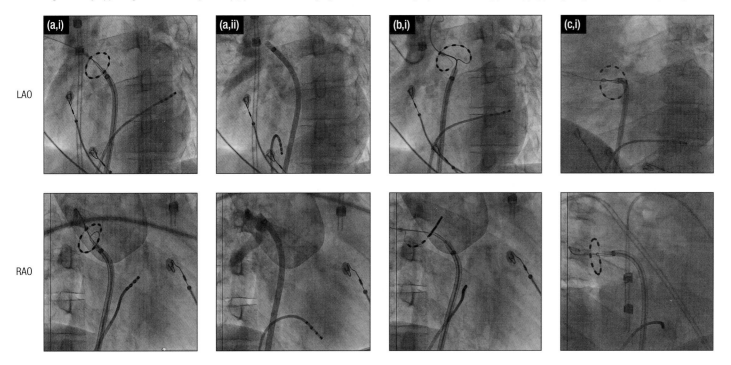

Targeting Pulmonary Veins: The Right Inferior Pulmonary Vein

- Usually, the right inferior pulmonary vein (RIPV) has a horizontal take-off from the LA wall

- There are three options available for moving the steerable sheath or the PVAC onto the RIPV (**Figure 12**):

  1. From the RSPV, curve the PVAC or sheath and pull and rotate it counter-clockwise to access the vein from above

  2. Point the PVAC towards the LSPV, make a sharp curve, extend the guidewire, and pull the catheter down and backwards onto the vein antrum (**Figure 13a**)

  3. Point the PVAC/sheath towards the LIPV, make a 90° curve, and turn it clockwise to access the RIPV from the side (**Figure 13b**)

- Steerable sheath: use sheath steerability only for stable positioning perpendicular to the wall (**Figure 13c**). The PVAC can remain straight and may be rotated freely

- Extending the distal end of the catheter array below the inferior rim of the RIPV and rotating it counter-clockwise will bring about inferior RIPV isolation away from the ostium (**Figure 13d**)

- Nonsteerable sheath: the shaft of the PVAC should be curved at an angle of 90° to the wall. The guidewire needs to be inserted deeper into the RIPV because rotation will tend to force the catheter out. The array of the catheter should be positioned on the lower edge of the vein to enable it to be extended for improved contact at the lower part of the PV

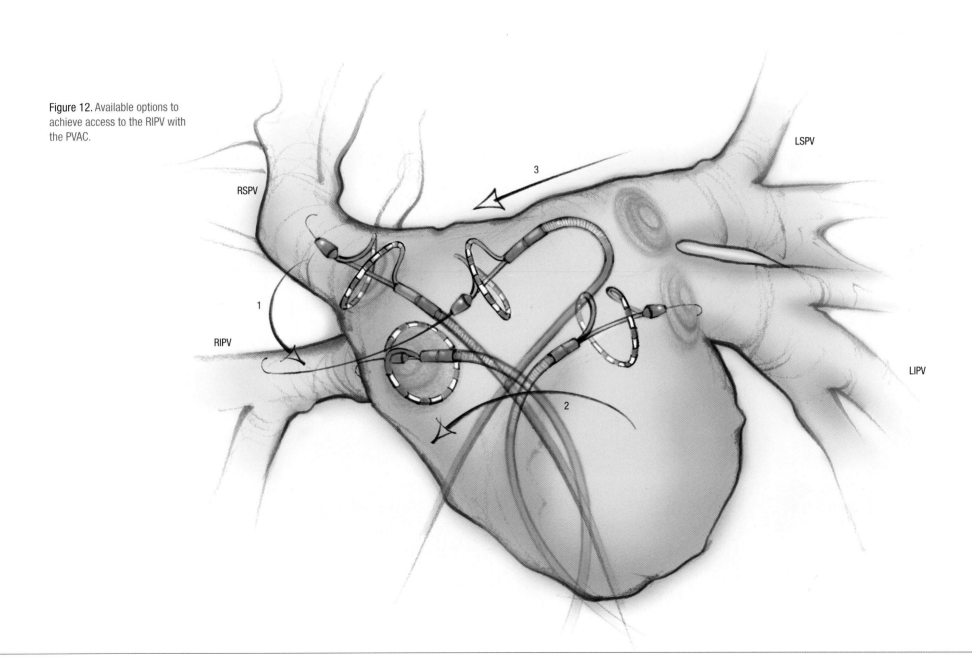

Figure 12. Available options to achieve access to the RIPV with the PVAC.

RSPV

LSPV

RIPV

LIPV

1

2

3

Figure 13. Techniques to cannulate the RIPV. The PVAC is pointed towards the LSPV, then (a,i) a sharp curve is made and the catheter is pulled down and backwards onto the RIPV antrum (a,ii). Alternatively, (b,i) the PVAC points to the LIPV, and (b,ii) by clockwise rotation provides lateral access to the RIPV.

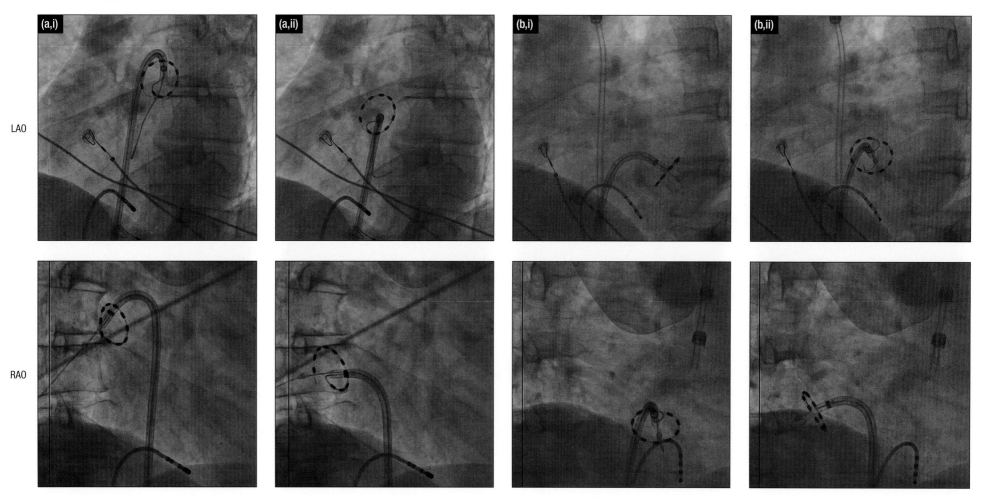

Figure 13. (c) Sheath steerability is used for stable positioning perpendicular to the wall, and (d) counter-clockwise rotation of the PVAC while extending the distal end of the array below the inferior rim for inferior RIPV isolation.

LAO

RAO

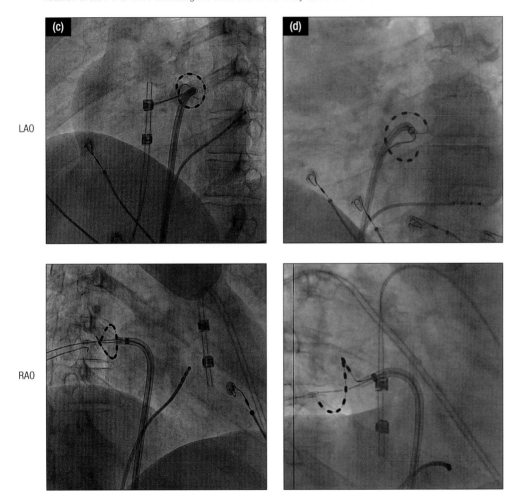

Confirmation of Isolation

PV potential mapping is employed post-ablation to confirm whether or not isolation has been achieved:

- Extend the distal end of the PVAC array and push the catheter into the PV with a clockwise rotation so that the spiral array is (partially) inside the ostium (*see* **Figure 6c**). By rotating the array, an absence of local potentials or isolated ectopy may be confirmed (**Figure 14**)

- When there is doubt about remaining potentials then the following corrective options are available:

  1. During CS pacing from a left lateral position, an absence of potentials can be verified in left-sided PVs (**Figure 14**) (this will be explained in **Chapter 6**)

  2. Pacing from the PVAC within the PV may show PV capture with exit block and perpetuation of sinus rhythm outside the PV (this will be explained in **Chapters 6** and **7**)

  3. Pacing from specific sites inside the LA or LAA around individual PV ostia may distinguish local potentials from far-field potentials (this will be explained in **Chapters 6** and **7**)

  4. Pharmacological challenges using isoproterenol or adenosine may reveal failed isolation (this will be explained in **Chapter 7**)

  5. Use a standard circular mapping catheter to verify the signals (this will be explained in **Chapter 5**)

  6. Voltage mapping with a three-dimensional mapping system may help to determine successful ablation in the PV antra

Figure 14. Ablation and verification of LSPV isolation. (a) Local PV potentials (∗) before ablation, and (b) an absence of PV potentials during CS pacing with isolated ectopy (∗) in the LSPV.

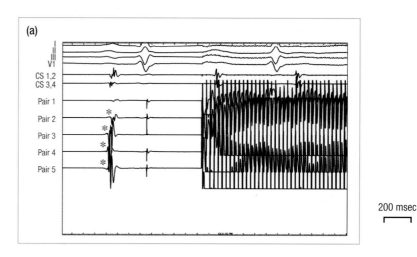

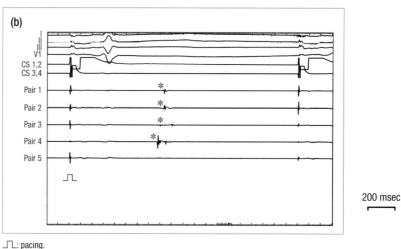

⎍: pacing.

Conclusion

- Use (biplane) fluoroscopy of the PVs to determine anatomical landmarks

- "Work with the catheter to make it work" by using all options available for the steerable sheath, the PVAC shaft, extending and rotating the array, and different positions of the guidewire

- Apply pressure to increase contact and temperature but avoid ablation inside the vein

- Map PV potentials before and after ablation to facilitate verification of electrical isolation by a variety of established pacing maneuvers and pharmacological challenges

4 | The Electrode and the Electrogram

This chapter describes the differences in electrode size and inter-electrode distance between conventional circular mapping catheters and the Pulmonary Vein Ablation Catheter (PVAC). The possible impact on bipolar electrogram morphology is discussed. Finally, representative tracings are shown of left atrial bipolar electrograms that have been recorded simultaneously using both mapping devices.

Learning Objectives

> *To acknowledge the comparative differences between conventional circular mapping catheters and the PVAC*

> *To appreciate that the PVAC has 10 electrodes that can be used both for ablation and mapping*

> *To understand that the electrodes of the PVAC can reliably record atrial bipolar electrograms*

> *To understand the effect of wave front propagation and the difference in electrode size and inter-electrode distance on the recording of bipolar electrograms (PVAC versus conventional mapping catheters)*

> *To appreciate how the PVAC can be used to reliably record and discriminate between pulmonary vein potentials*

The PVAC: Just Another Circular Mapping Catheter?

As with most conventional circular mapping catheters (CMCs; Lasso™, Biosense Webster Inc., Diamond Bar, CA, USA; Optima™, St. Jude Medical Inc., St. Paul, MN, USA), the PVAC is a 10-pole circular catheter with a maximum diameter of approximately 25 mm (**Figure 1**). Therefore, by nature of its design, the PVAC should be an adequate tool for the assessment of pulmonary vein (PV) isolation.

Figure 1. Characteristics of (a) CMCs, and (b) the PVAC.

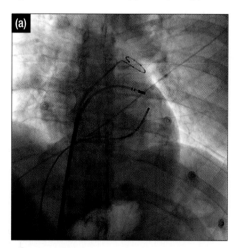 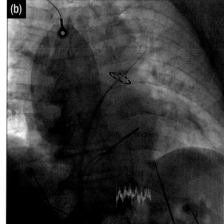

(a) Conventional CMCs
- 10-Pole (or 14- or 20-pole) circular catheter
- Fixed or variable (maximum diameter 25 mm)
- Need for ablation catheter

(b) PVAC
- 10-Pole circular catheter
- Maximum diameter 25 mm
- Mapping and ablation

Direct Comparison of Electrode Characteristics

Conventional CMCs have an electrode size of 1 × 1 mm with an inter-electrode distance of 7–8 mm (**Figure 2**); the PVAC has electrodes with a length of 3 mm, a diameter of 1.5 mm, and an inter-electrode space of 3 mm.

Differences in electrode design may have implications for the characteristics of recorded bipolar electrograms (Bip EGMs; *see next section*).

Figure 2. Comparative electrode characteristics between (a) conventional CMCs, and (b) the PVAC.

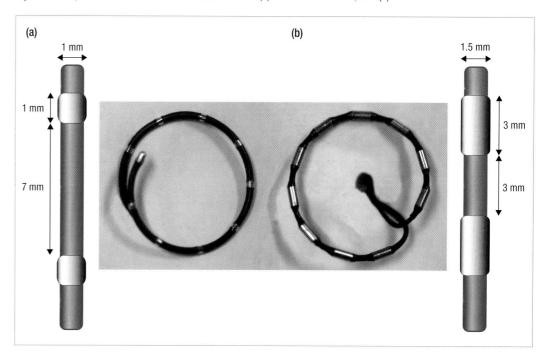

Bipolar Electrograms Recorded With the PVAC may be More Smoothened in Parallel Propagation

As a consequence of the PVAC having a large electrode size (3 mm), unipolar electrograms (Uni EGMs) recorded with the PVAC are expected to have a waveform that has a smaller amplitude and is less steep compared with that seen on using a conventional CMC (**Figure 3**).

The resulting Bip EGM recorded with the PVAC is expected to have a waveform that has a smaller amplitude, is more smoothened, and has less detail. This is particularly the case if the wave front travels in parallel with the longitudinal axis of the electrodes.

Figure 3. Differences in waveform between (a) conventional CMCs, and (b) the PVAC.

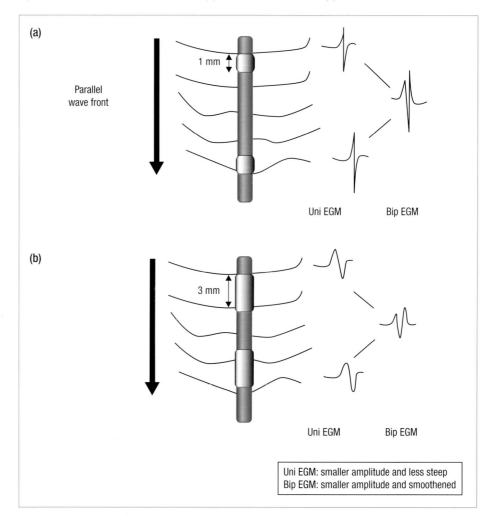

(a)

1 mm

Parallel wave front

Uni EGM   Bip EGM

(b)

3 mm

Uni EGM   Bip EGM

Uni EGM: smaller amplitude and less steep
Bip EGM: smaller amplitude and smoothened

Bipolar Electrograms Recorded With the PVAC in Perpendicular Propagation

During mapping for PV isolation, the wave front (sinus rhythm or pacing) is expected to travel perpendicular to the longitudinal axis of the electrodes (**Figure 4**). Because of this, the difference in amplitude and detail in Bip EGMs (**Figure 5**) recorded with other CMCs is not expected to be as small as that obtained with the PVAC.

Figure 4. PVAC: perpendicular travel of the wave front.

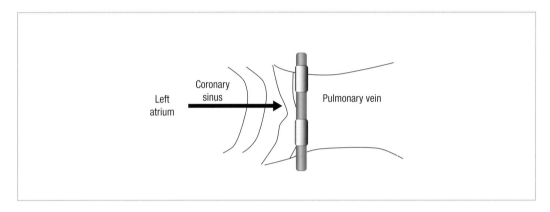

Figure 5. Bip EGMs show that compared with (a) conventional CMCs, (b) the PVAC has comparatively small differences in amplitude.

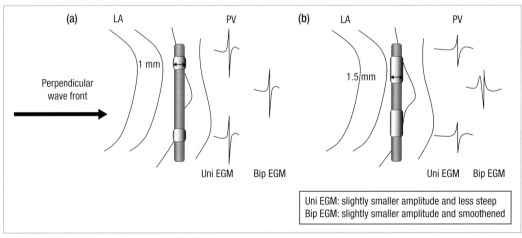

LA: left atrium.

Comparison of Bipolar Left Atrial Pulmonary Vein Electrograms Recorded With a Conventional Circular Mapping Catheter and the PVAC

Figure 6a and **b** show the fluoroscopic position of the catheters in the right superior pulmonary vein (RSPV); **Figure 6c** shows the corresponding atriography (obtained after nonselective left atrial injection of contrast medium after adenosine).

Figure 6. (a) Position of the PVAC within the RSPV, (b) similar position of a CMC, and (c) nonselective atriography.

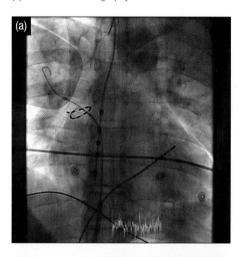
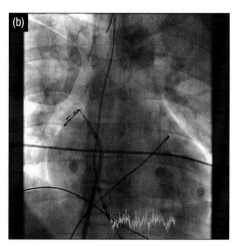
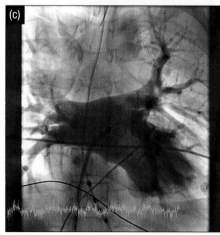

The Bip EGM recorded in the RSPV with the PVAC (**Figure 7a**) has a waveform with a slightly smaller amplitude, is more smoothened, and has less detail compared with that recorded utilizing a conventional CMC in the same fluoroscopic position (**Figure 7b**).

The Bip EGM recorded with the PVAC, however, still reveals all critical components (far-field and PV potential) of the left atrial pulmonary vein (LA-PV) electrogram.

Figure 7. Mapping comparison of Bip EGMs recorded in the RSPV between (a) the PVAC and (b) a conventional CMC.

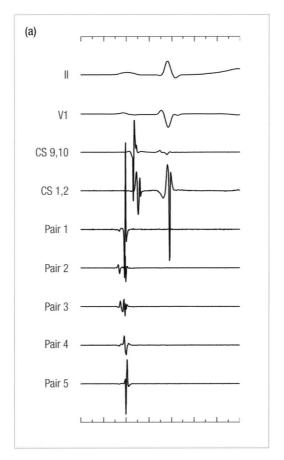
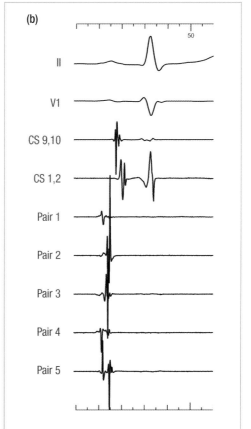

Figure 8a and **b** show the fluoroscopic position of the catheters in the left superior pulmonary vein (LSPV); **Figure 8c** shows the corresponding selective PV angiography.

Differences can be observed in electrogram characteristics recorded by the PVAC (**Figure 9a**) and a conventional CMC (**Figure 9b**).

The Bip EGM recorded with the PVAC (fluoroscopically torqued within the LSPV) has a slightly smaller amplitude and is less detailed compared with that of the electrogram recorded utilizing a conventional CMC.

The PVAC Bip EGM, however, still reveals all critical components of the LA-PV electrogram during pacing at the distal coronary sinus. Furthermore, because of the nature of its design, the PVAC allows for proximal to distal assessment of PV conduction.

Figure 8. (a) Torqued position of the PVAC within the LSPV, (b) mapping position of a CMC, and (c) selective angiography.

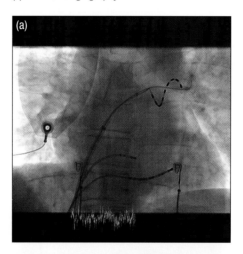
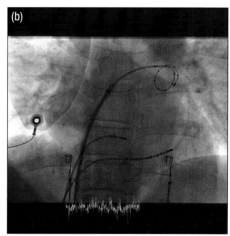
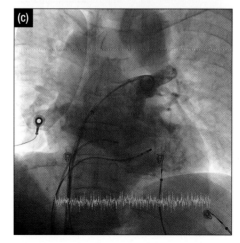

Figure 9. Mapping comparison of Bip EGMs recorded in the LSPV between (a) the PVAC and (b) a conventional CMC.

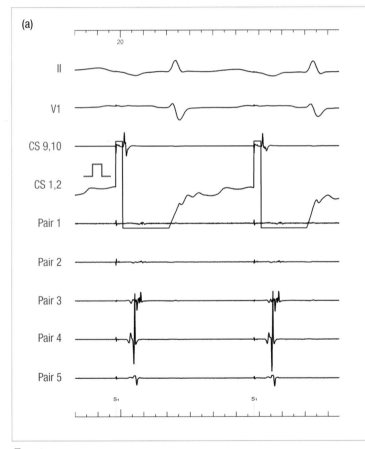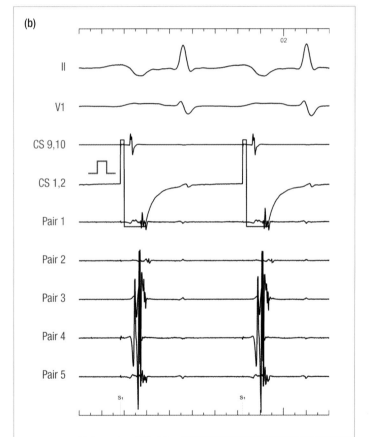

⌐⌐: pacing.

Recommended Settings for Recording High-Quality Bipolar Electrograms During Pulmonary Vein Isolation

- The PVAC can be used to record high-quality Bip EGMs and allows for differentiation of far-field and PV potentials

- Recording of Bip EGMs with the PVAC can be performed using:

  - Five PVAC traces

  - Amplification (Bard EP: gain 16; Prucka EP: gain 5,000)

  - Filter settings:

    - High-pass: 100 Hz

    - Low-pass: 500 Hz

Conclusion

- Compared with conventional CMCs, the PVAC has 10 electrodes that can be used both for mapping and ablation of PVs

- The PVAC can reliably record atrial Bip EGMs and can be used to reliably assess the absence or presence of PV potentials

5 | How to Assess Pulmonary Vein Isolation Using the PVAC and the Coronary Sinus Catheter

This chapter describes how to assess electrical isolation of the pulmonary veins using
the Pulmonary Vein Ablation Catheter (PVAC) and coronary sinus catheter only.

Learning Objectives

> *To find out how to use the PVAC as a mapping tool during both sinus rhythm and atrial fibrillation*

> *To acknowledge how pulmonary vein potentials can be reliably mapped with the PVAC (a circular mapping catheter was used for educational purposes in order to confirm pulmonary vein isolation and prove the diagnostic accuracy of the PVAC)*

> *To appreciate that the PVAC can be used as a stand-alone catheter (for mapping and ablation) without the need for a conventional circular mapping catheter*

Ablation Using the PVAC: Proof of Concept

The proof of concept of PVAC ablation is shown in **Figure 1**.

After positioning the PVAC at the proximal ostium of the left inferior pulmonary vein (LIPV), a circular mapping catheter (CMC) was maneuvered past the PVAC and positioned more distally within the same vein (**Figure 1a**).

Figure 1. PVAC ablation: proof of concept. **(a)** Positioning of the PVAC and a CMC in the LIPV.

At baseline, the CMC revealed typical pulmonary vein (PV) potentials (**Figure 1b**). After delivery of 1 min of radiofrequency (RF) energy ablation and without moving the CMC, the PV was proven to be isolated (**Figure 1c**).

Figure 1. (b) Before, and (c) after RF energy ablation.

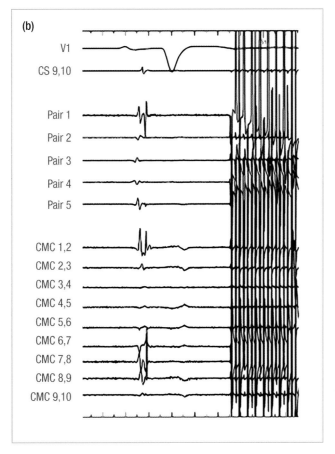

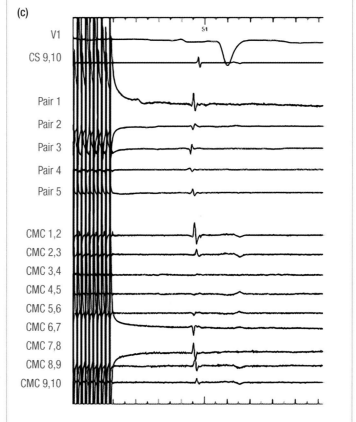

100 msec

How to Map With the PVAC

Proximal PVAC ablation is performed by positioning the PVAC at the ostium of the left superior pulmonary vein (LSPV; **Figure 2a**) and guiding it by selective PV angiography, nonselective atriography, or three-dimensional rotational angiography. Distal PVAC mapping (**Figure 2b**) is performed by torqueing the PVAC more distally within the LSPV.

To reliably assess PV isolation with the PVAC, distal PVAC mapping can be performed:

- Both at baseline (electrogram templates before any delivery of RF energy) and after ablation

- Respecting the same anatomical position (importance of fluoroscopic references)

- During sinus rhythm and pacing at the proximal coronary sinus (CSP) for right PVs, or at the distal coronary sinus (CSD) for left PVs.

Figure 2. (a) Ablation, and (b) mapping of the LSPV with the PVAC.

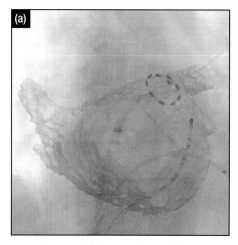 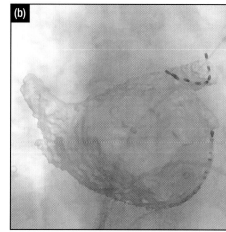

Proximal PVAC ablation is performed by positioning the PVAC at the ostium of the LIPV (**Figure 3a**) and guiding it by selective PV angiography, nonselective atriography, or three-dimensional rotational angiography.

Distal PVAC mapping (**Figure 3b**) is performed by torqueing the PVAC more distally within the LIPV.

Figure 3. (a) Ablation, and (b) mapping of the LIPV with the PVAC.

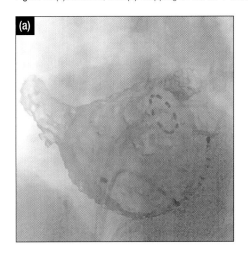 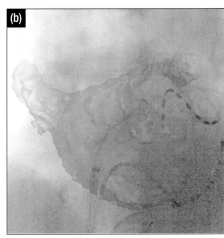

Mapping of the Left Superior Pulmonary Vein Before and After Ablation: Isolation

Figure 4 shows the fluoroscopic position of the PVAC in the LSPV (**a**), and the corresponding selective angiography (**b**).

Figure 5 shows the bipolar electrograms recorded by the PVAC within the LSPV during sinus rhythm and pacing at the CSD (ie, CS 1,2) both before (**a**) and after (**b**) proximal ablation (4 min of RF energy).

Before RF energy ablation, distal mapping with the PVAC revealed a fusion of the far-field (∗) and high-frequency PV potentials (↓). During pacing at the CSD the far-field and PV potentials are separated to a greater degree (**Figure 5a**).

After RF ablation (**Figure 5b**), PVAC mapping within the LSPV revealed residual potentials (∗) suggestive of far-field signals from the left atrial appendage (LAA) during sinus rhythm. Pacing at the CSD revealed a single, low-gradient potential.

Without having a template at baseline (which unmasked the far-field and PV potentials) it would be difficult to verify isolation. Electrical isolation was confirmed by mapping with a conventional CMC (*see next section*).

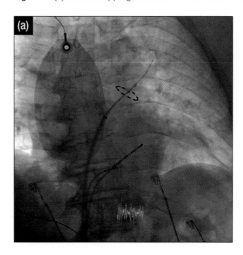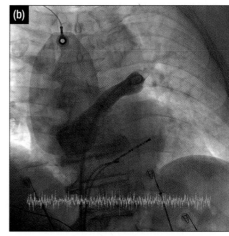

Figure 4. (a) Distal mapping of the LSPV with the PVAC, and (b) selective angiography of the LSPV.

Figure 5. Mapping of the LSPV (a) before, and (b) after RF energy ablation.

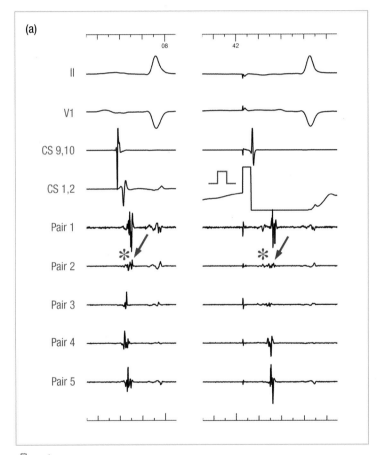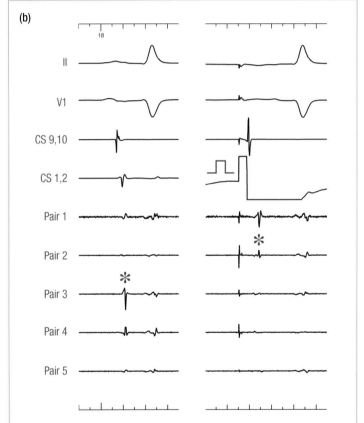

⌐⌐: pacing.

Confirmation of Left Superior Pulmonary Vein Isolation

In this case (the same as described above), **Figure 6** shows the positioning of a CMC, and **Figure 7** confirms the absence of PV potentials in the LSPV on using a conventional CMC after PVAC mapping and ablation.

Figure 6. Fluoroscopic position of a conventional CMC in the LSPV.

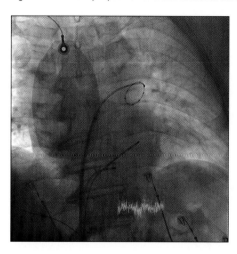

Figure 7. Confirmation of PV isolation using a conventional CMC (a) before, and (b) after RF energy ablation.

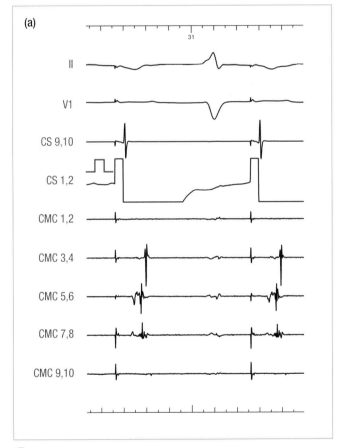
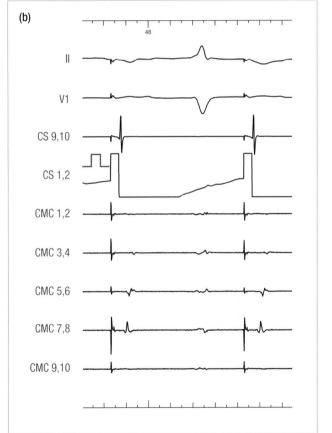

⌐L : pacing.

Mapping of the Right Inferior Pulmonary Vein Before and After Ablation: Isolation

Figure 8 shows the fluoroscopic position of the PVAC in the right inferior pulmonary vein (RIPV) (**a**), and the corresponding selective angiography (**b**).

Figure 9 shows distal PVAC mapping within the RIPV during sinus rhythm and pacing at CSP (ie, CS 9,10) both before (**a**) and after (**b**) proximal ablation (2 min of RF energy ablation).

After RF energy ablation (**Figure 9b**), PVAC mapping within the RIPV still revealed potentials (∗) during sinus rhythm, but with a low amplitude and a biphasic pattern (RS and qR). The potentials have a relatively late timing (>40 msec from the onset of the P-wave).

Without having a template at baseline (**Figure 9a**), it would be difficult to determine isolation. Compared with baseline, however, the high-frequency potentials (↓) seem to have disappeared after ablation. This is especially clear during pacing at the CSP, which resulted in apparent differentiation between the far-field (posterior wall of the left atrium [LA]) and the PV potentials at baseline.

These findings strongly suggest that there is electrical isolation with a residual far-field signal from the posterior wall of the LA. Electrical isolation was confirmed by mapping with a conventional CMC (*see next section*).

Figure 8. (a) Distal mapping of the RIPV with the PVAC, and (b) selective angiography of the RIPV.

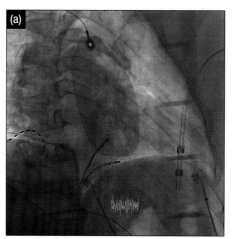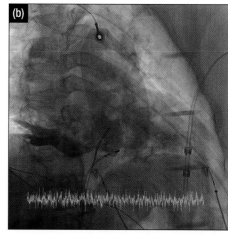

Figure 9. PVAC mapping of the RIPV (a) before, and (b) after RF energy ablation.

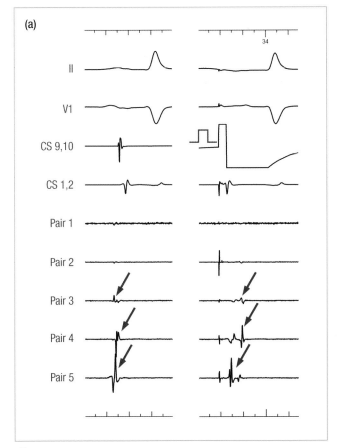
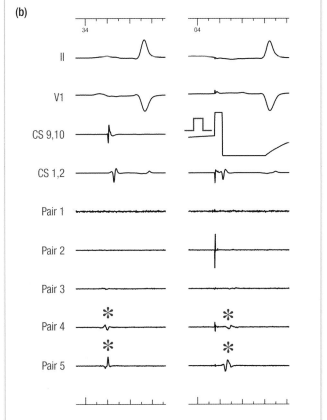

⎍ : pacing.

Confirmation of Right Inferior Pulmonary Vein Isolation

In this case (the same as described above), **Figure 10** shows the positioning of the CMC, and **Figure 11** confirms the absence of PV potentials within the RIPV on using a conventional CMC before and after PVAC mapping and ablation.

After ablation, pacing at the posterior wall (via an extra transseptal 4-mm catheter) advanced all potentials to within 20 msec of the stimulus signal (not shown). This provided a strong confirmation of electrical isolation.

Figure 10. Fluoroscopic position of a conventional CMC in the RIPV.

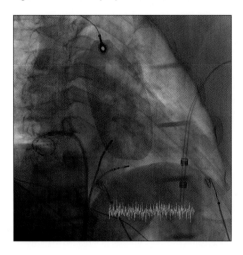

Figure 11. Mapping of the RIPV using a conventional CMC (a) before, and (b) after RF energy ablation.

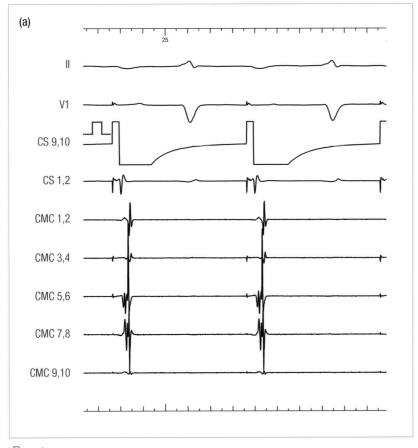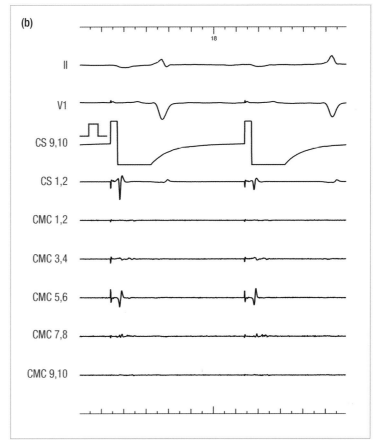

⊓ : pacing.

Mapping of the Left Superior Pulmonary Vein Before and After Ablation: Is this Vein Isolated?

Figure 12 shows the position of the PVAC within the LSPV (**a**), and the corresponding selective angiography (**b**).

Figure 13 shows distal PVAC mapping within the LSPV during pacing in the CSD at baseline (**a**) and after (**b**) ablation.

After RF ablation (**Figure 13b**), PVAC mapping continued to reveal a high-frequency and large-amplitude potential on electrode pair 4 (∗). Despite this, the potential most likely reflects a far-field signal from the LAA because: (i) during pacing at the CSD, a potential with a stimulus-to-atrium interval of 60–80 msec is suggestive of LAA, (ii) electrode pair 4 faces the LAA, and (iii) the high-frequency PV potentials present at baseline have disappeared (↓).

Differential pacing at the LAA could be useful in this case (not performed).

Electrical isolation was confirmed by mapping with a CMC (*see next section*).

Figure 12. (a) Distal mapping of the LSPV with the PVAC, and (b) selective angiography of the LSPV.

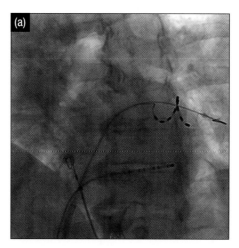
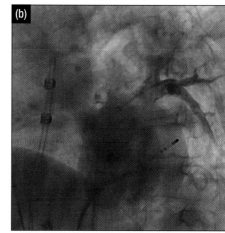

Figure 13. PVAC mapping of the LSPV during pacing at the CSD (a) before, and (b) after RF energy ablation.

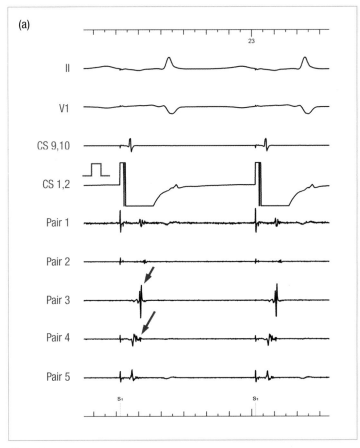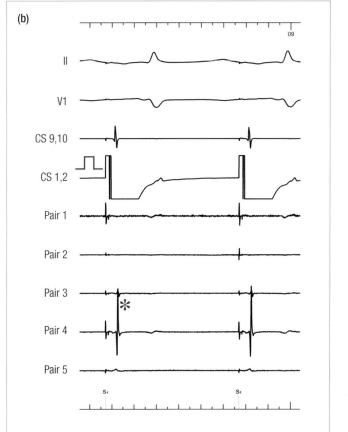

⊓: pacing.

Verification of Left Superior Pulmonary Vein Isolation

In this case (the same as described above), the absence of PV potentials within the LSPV was confirmed using a CMC before (**a**) and after (**b**) PVAC mapping and ablation (**Figure 14**).

Pacing at the LAA (via an extra transseptal 4-mm catheter) advanced the potential to within 40 msec of the stimulus signal (not shown). This provided a strong confirmation of electrical isolation.

Figure 14. Confirmation of the absence of PV potentials within the LSPV using a conventional CMC (a) before, and (b) after PVAC ablation.

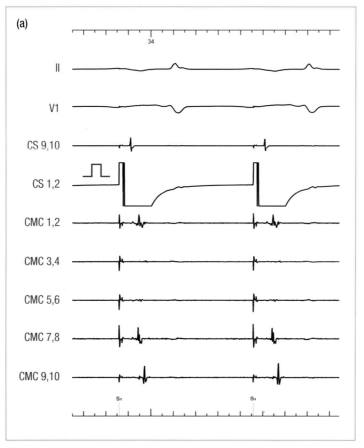
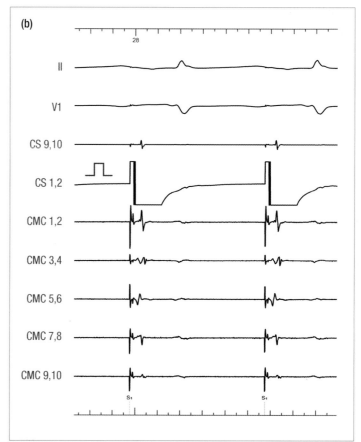

100 msec

⊓: pacing.

Mapping of the Right Superior Pulmonary Vein Before and After Ablation: Bidirectional Isolation

Figure 15 shows distal PVAC mapping within the right superior pulmonary vein (RSPV) during sinus rhythm at baseline (**a**) and after (**b**) proximal ablation.

After 3 min of RF energy ablation (**Figure 15b**), PVAC mapping revealed automaticity (↓) within the RSPV with residual far-field potentials (most likely originating from the superior vena cava [SVC], *) during sinus rhythm (ie, bidirectional block). After this, the baseline recordings (showing far-field and PV potentials before RF energy delivery) were not needed to make a correct diagnosis.

Figure 15. PVAC mapping within the RSPV during sinus rhythm at (a) baseline, and (b) after proximal ablation.

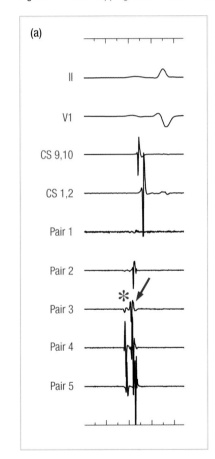
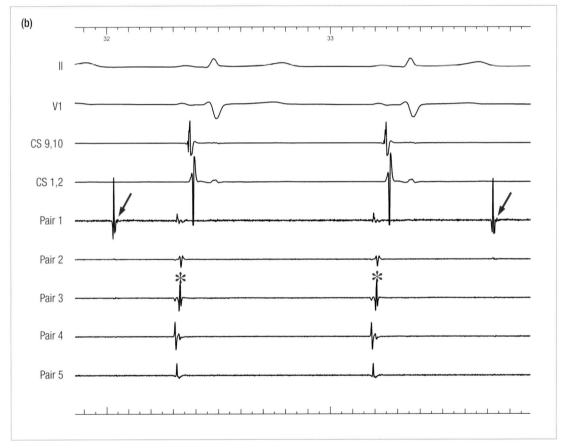

Mapping of Residual "Tiny" Potentials Within the Right Inferior Pulmonary Vein After Ablation

Figure 16 shows the fluoroscopic position of the PVAC in the RIPV (**a**), and the corresponding selective angiography (**b**).

Figure 17 shows distal PVAC mapping within the RIPV during sinus rhythm at baseline (**a**) and after ablation (**b**). Before any RF energy delivery, the PVAC electrograms recorded within the RIPV revealed far-field (∗) and PV potentials (↓, pair 1).

After five RF energy applications, distal PVAC mapping within the RIPV revealed only small residual fractionated signals (∗, pairs 3 and 4). Also, because of their early timing (occurring before CS activation during sinus rhythm) despite prior RF ablation, they were interpreted as being far-field signals. Therefore, PVAC ablation was stopped.

Figure 16. (a) Distal mapping of the RIPV with the PVAC, and (b) selective angiography.

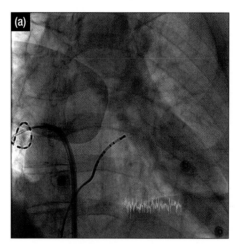
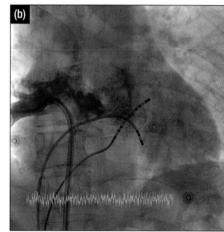

Figure 17. PVAC mapping within the RIPV during sinus rhythm at (a) baseline, and (b) after proximal ablation.

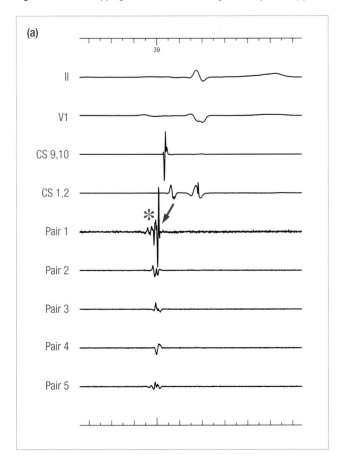
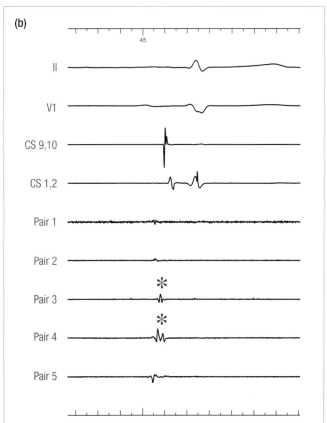

Residual Pulmonary Vein Potentials Within the Right Inferior Pulmonary Vein on Using a Circular Mapping Catheter

In this case (the same as described above), after presumed isolation, PV potentials (↓, pair 3) and late fragmented potentials (pair 4) were still revealed on using a conventional CMC (**Figure 18a**).

The PVAC was repositioned at the RIPV antrum and gap potentials were observed at the posterior wall (not shown). With continued PVAC ablation these PV potentials could also be eliminated (**Figure 18b**).

The initial mapping error (*see previous section*) was most likely to be related to the difficult positioning of the PVAC within the RIPV because of the proximal branching of this vein.

Other mapping maneuvers (such as exit pacing from the PVAC or adding an LA pacing catheter for differential pacing) may help (*see* **Chapters 6** and **7**).

Following this, it could be argued that "distal" PVAC mapping could have been performed more proficiently given the persistence of residual fractionated potentials at the end of ablation (*see previous section*). On the other hand, this is a *post-hoc* discussion of a typical real-life case. It accentuates the need for thorough mapping to confirm PV isolation.

Figure 18. Mapping with a conventional CMC. (a) Residual PV potentials within the RIPV after PVAC ablation, and (b) isolation is finally proven after continued PVAC ablation.

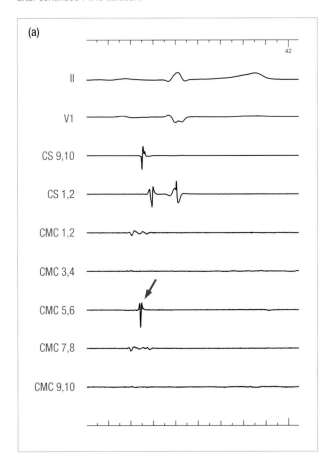
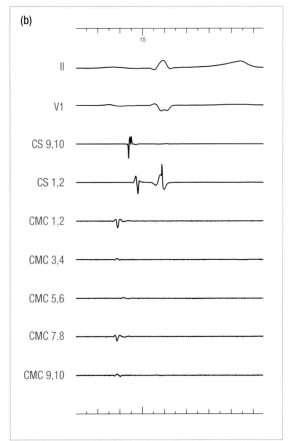

Mapping of the Left Inferior Pulmonary Vein Before and After Ablation During Atrial Fibrillation: Increasing the Degree of Entrance Block

Figure 19 shows the fluoroscopic position of the PVAC in the LIPV.

Figure 20 shows distal PVAC mapping within the LIPV during atrial fibrillation (AF) at baseline (**a**) and after (**b**) proximal PVAC ablation.

Before any RF energy delivery (**Figure 20a**), bipolar PVAC electrograms revealed far-field (∗) and dominant high-frequency (↓) PV potentials. The AF cycle length of the PV potential is 160 msec.

After two proximal applications (**Figure 20b**), distal mapping revealed a marked increase in the AF cycle length of the PV potential (280 msec, pairs 1 and 5) suggesting an increasing degree of entrance block (↓). The unchanged AF cycle length of the signals from pairs 2 to 4 suggests that these bipoles record far-field signals from the anterior LA (∗).

As a consequence of residual LA-PV conduction, the PVAC was withdrawn to the ostium of the LIPV to continue ablation (*see next section*).

Figure 19. Distal mapping of the LIPV with the PVAC.

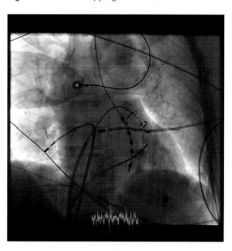

Figure 20. PVAC mapping within the LIPV during AF at (a) baseline, and (b) after proximal ablation.

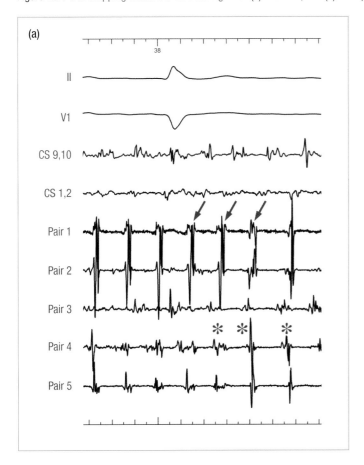
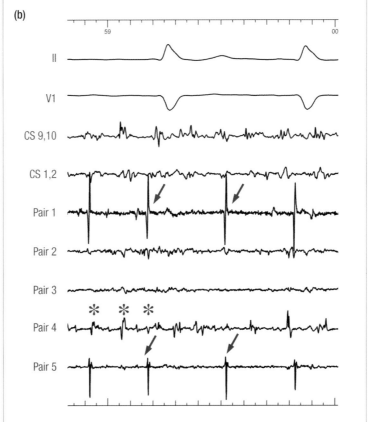

100 msec

Mapping of the Left Inferior Pulmonary Vein After Ablation During Atrial Fibrillation: Isolation

In this case (the same as described above), after continued ablation, **Figure 21** showed that distal PVAC mapping within the LIPV revealed only residual far-field signals during AF (unchanged cycle length, *), suggesting electrical isolation.

After electrical cardioversion (**Figure 21b**), distal PVAC mapping revealed a single, low-frequency signal with no apparent delay (*). Because the timing during pacing at the CSD (ie, CS 1,2) was compatible with the far-field signal from the anterior LA, isolation was presumed and PVAC ablation at the LIPV was stopped.

Electrical isolation was confirmed by mapping with a conventional CMC (*see next section*).

Figure 21. PVAC mapping within the LIPV after ablation (a) during AF, and (b) after cardioversion.

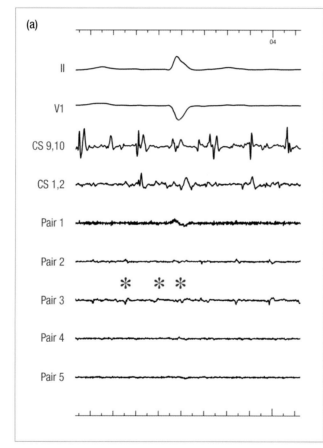
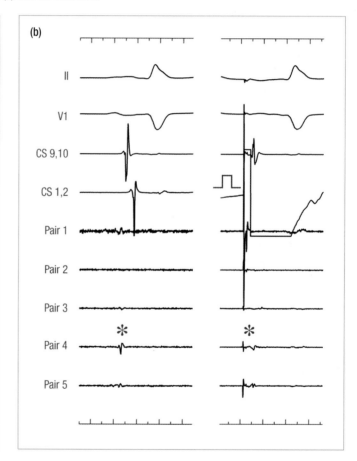

⊓: pacing.

100 msec

Confirmation of Left Inferior Pulmonary Vein Isolation

In this case (the same as described above), electrical isolation of the LIPV was confirmed using a conventional CMC (**Figure 22**) before (**Figure 23a**) and after (**Figure 23b**) PVAC mapping and ablation. Pacing was performed at the CS 1,2 pair.

Figure 22. Fluoroscopic position of a conventional CMC within the LIPV.

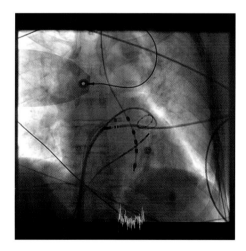

Figure 23. Confirmation of electrical isolation of the LIPV using a conventional CMC during pacing at the CSD (a) before, and (b) after PVAC ablation.

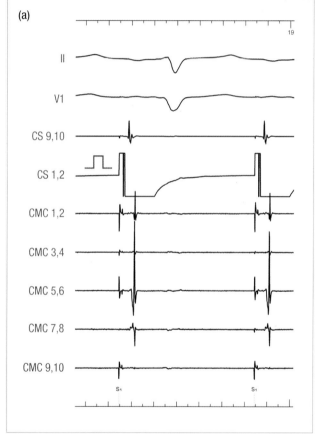
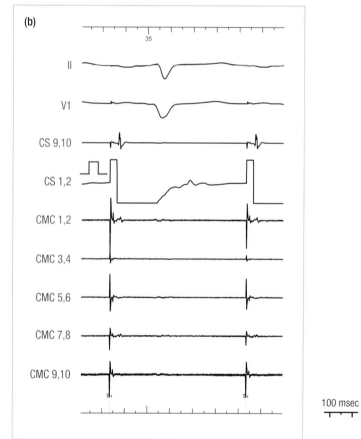

⎍ : pacing.

100 msec

Mapping of the Right Superior Pulmonary Vein Before and After Ablation During Atrial Fibrillation: Is this Vein Isolated?

Figure 24 shows the mapping position of the PVAC within the RSPV.

Figure 25 shows the bipolar electrograms recorded with the PVAC during AF at baseline (**a**) and after (**b**) proximal PVAC ablation.

Before any RF energy delivery (**Figure 25a**), bipolar PVAC electrograms revealed dominant high-frequency PV potentials (↓) in all pairs. The AF cycle length of the PV potentials is 170 msec.

After three proximal applications, distal PVAC mapping (**Figure 25b**) revealed a marked increase in the AF cycle length in between the sharp potentials (↓; to >400 msec in pairs 1 and 5), suggesting an increased degree of entrance block in the remaining PV sleeves.

The catheter was withdrawn to the ostium of the RSPV to continue more proximal ablation (*see next section*).

Figure 24. Fluoroscopic position of the PVAC within the RSPV.

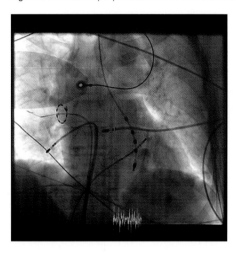

Figure 25. PVAC mapping within the RSPV during AF (a) at baseline, and (b) after proximal PVAC ablation.

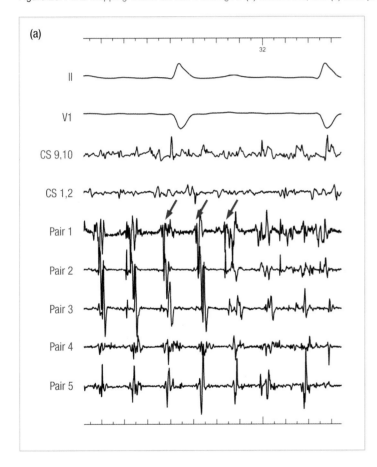
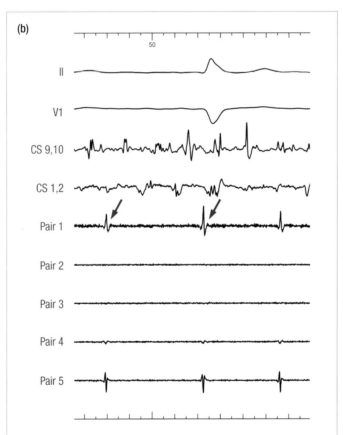

Mapping of the Right Superior Pulmonary Vein After Ablation: Far Field from the Superior Vena Cava During Atrial Fibrillation

In this case (the same as described above), despite additional proximal ablation, the PVAC still revealed residual sharp signals (pairs 1 and 5) with a cycle length of approximately 400 msec within the RSPV (∗; **Figure 26**). Therefore, the CS catheter was positioned at the postero-septal wall of the SVC. The bipolar electrogram recorded at the SVC revealed sharp and high-amplitude signals (↓). Clearly, the residual signals on the PVAC reflected the far-field signals from the SVC.

After electrical cardioversion, distal PVAC mapping confirmed electrical isolation during sinus rhythm with an idio-PV rhythm indicating bidirectional block (not shown).

Figure 26. PVAC mapping of the RSPV during AF after ablation. The tip of the CS catheter was positioned within the SVC.

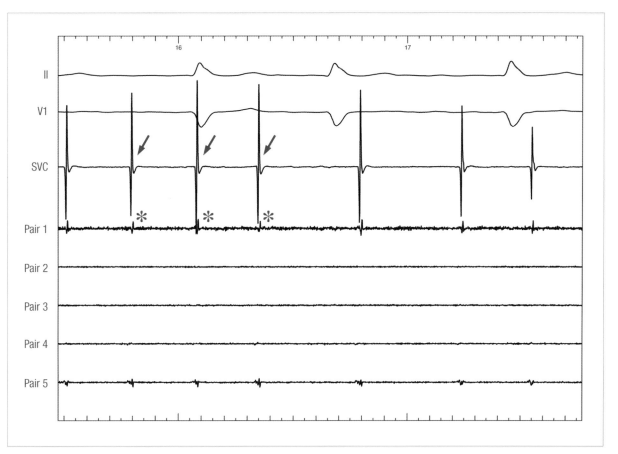

Mapping of Residual Potential Within the Left Inferior Pulmonary Vein During Atrial Fibrillation

Figure 27 shows the fluoroscopic position of the PVAC in the LIPV (**a**), and the corresponding left atriography (**b**).

Figure 28 shows the distal PVAC mapping within the LIPV during AF at baseline (**a**) and after (**b**) proximal PVAC ablation.

Before any RF energy delivery (**Figure 28a**), bipolar PVAC electrograms revealed high-frequency PV signals (↓, pairs 3 and 5).

After three proximal applications, distal PVAC mapping (**Figure 28b**) revealed only low-amplitude signals consistent with far-field (∗) signals from the anterior LA and the ventricle.

As a consequence of presumed isolation, ablation was continued in the other PVs. Later, electrical cardioversion was performed to verify isolation (*see next section*).

Figure 27. (a) Distal mapping of the LIPV with the PVAC, and (b) nonselective atriography after adenosine injection.

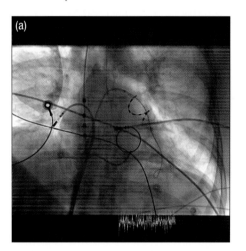
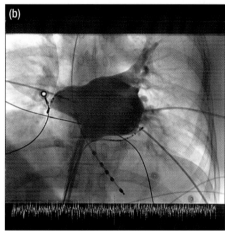

Figure 28. PVAC mapping within the LIPV during AF (a) at baseline, and (b) after proximal PVAC ablation.

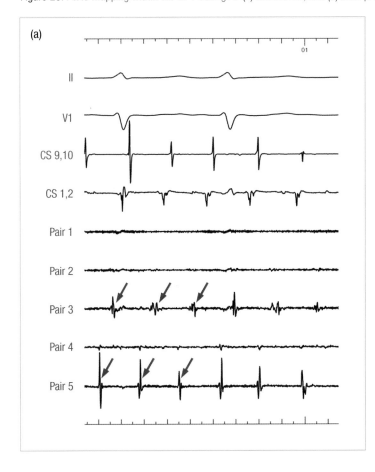
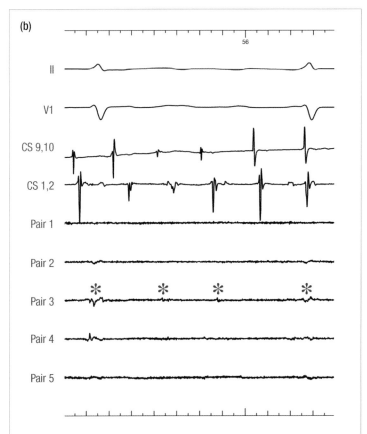

Mapping of the Left Inferior Pulmonary Vein After Electrical Cardioversion: Residual Pulmonary Vein Potentials

In the same case as described above, despite presumed isolation during AF, after cardioversion distal PVAC mapping within the LIPV still revealed a sharp potential with late timing (↓, pair 5; **Figure 29a**). This was strongly suggestive of residual PV potentials.

Only after continued proximal ablation was isolation obtained (**Figure 29b**). Electrical isolation was confirmed by mapping with a conventional CMC (*see next section*).

These findings favor a strategy to verify PV isolation consistently during sinus rhythm after PVAC ablation during AF. It is likely that during AF the signal morphology and quality may vary markedly and PV potentials may be masked.

Figure 29. PVAC mapping within the LIPV (a) after electrical cardioversion, and (b) after continued PVAC ablation.

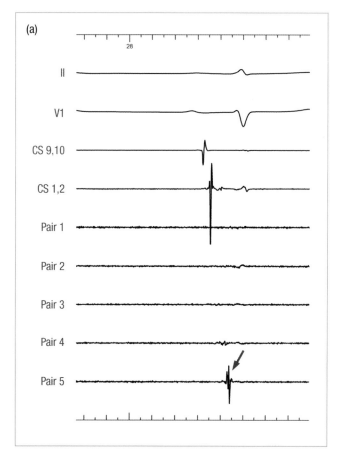
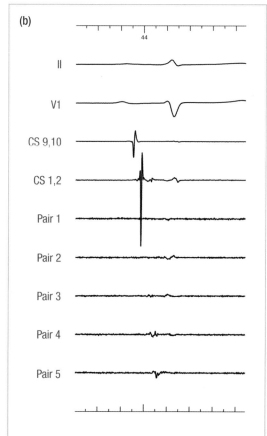

Mapping of the Left Superior Pulmonary Vein During Atrial Fibrillation and After Cardioversion

Distal PVAC mapping was carried out within the LSPV during AF at baseline (**Figure 30a**), and during sinus rhythm after proximal PVAC ablation (**Figure 30b**).

Before ablation, bipolar PVAC electrograms revealed high-frequency PV potentials during AF (↓; **Figure 30a**). Ablation was continued until distal PVAC mapping suggested PV isolation during AF (not shown).

Electrical cardioversion was performed to check isolation (**Figure 30b**). During pacing at the CSD, distal PVAC mapping still revealed high-frequency signals (∗). The timing was compatible with the far-field signal from the LAA. Pacing at the LAA (via an extra transseptal 4-mm catheter) advanced the potential to within 40 msec of the stimulus signal. This provided a strong confirmation of electrical isolation.

Electrical isolation was confirmed by mapping with a conventional CMC (not shown).

Figure 30. PVAC mapping within the LSPV during AF (a) at baseline, and (b) during sinus rhythm after proximal PVAC ablation.

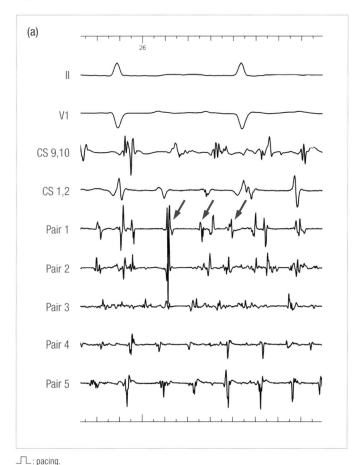

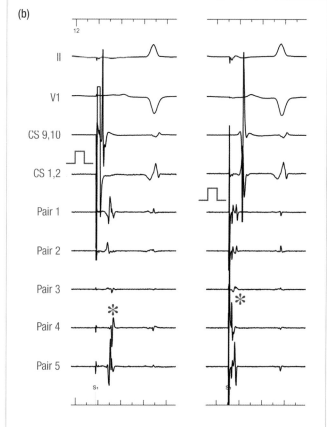

⊓: pacing.

100 msec

Conclusion

- The PVAC can be used to ablate, pace, and map isolation of the PVs

- To reliably assess PV isolation, distal PVAC mapping should be performed at baseline and after ablation, during both sinus rhythm and differential pacing

- When ablating during AF, isolation should be verified after cardioversion

6 | Differential Pacing Beyond the Coronary Sinus to Validate Isolation of the Pulmonary Vein

The Pulmonary Vein Ablation Catheter (PVAC) may record additional far-field signals when compared with a conventional circular mapping catheter because of the larger electrodes (3 mm vs. 1 mm) which can be used for ablation. Specifically, the electrical activation recorded on the PVAC can originate from multiple anatomical structures, such as a pulmonary vein, the left atrium, left atrial appendage, right atrium, etc, which may confound signal interpretation during sinus rhythm or coronary sinus pacing. This challenge can be resolved by pacing near the origin of the presumed far-field signal, eg, the left atrial appendage, to create an increased differentiation between signals coming from the anatomical structures. It should be noted that a far-field signal from the posterior left atrial wall may also show an increased delay during pacing of the anteriorally located left atrial appendage. This suggests that additional pacing maneuvers with the PVAC are feasible and can be used to separate far-field signals and to definitively confirm pulmonary vein isolation.

In this chapter the principle of differential pacing in the areas near the pulmonary veins is described. The aim is to provide simple techniques that use a single mapping or pacing catheter in addition to the PVAC. For this purpose, a steerable coronary sinus catheter is used in order to limit the number of femoral sheaths required.

Learning Objectives

> *To understand the principles of differential pacing*

> *To apply these principles to the differentiation of pulmonary vein signals from far-field atrial signals on using the PVAC*

Introduction

Isolation of a single pulmonary vein (PV) with the PVAC is not typically achieved from a single radiofrequency (RF) energy application, but rather as a result of several multipolar energy applications at different positions around the antrum and/or PV ostium. Results from a multicenter trial by Scharf et al in 2009 (*see Recommended Reading*) demonstrated that, on average, 6–10 RF energy applications were required per vein to achieve isolation. After delivering this typical number of lesions, the catheter operator may be interested in using additional maneuvers to discriminate the origin of residual electrogram signals as having an origin in the PVs or from a far-field source.

Differentiating the origin of these residual signals is important to reduce the number of unnecessary RF energy applications. Probatory RF energy delivery at the PV ostium uses a simple strategy that is known as "learning by burning," where near-field signals can be eliminated by RF energy ablation. However, far-field signals are not affected because the lesion does not affect the point of origin of the electrogram. This strategy may not only prolong the procedure and increase fluoroscopy exposure, but also carries a potential risk for complications due to unnecessary RF injury, such as PV stenosis or phrenic nerve palsy, and can deliver energy to the posterior left atrial (LA) wall. More importantly, if atrial far-field

signals are misinterpreted as PV signals, and do not disappear after probatory RF energy delivery, then the catheter operator may believe that the duty-cycled RF energy has been ineffective for achieving the procedural endpoint, and thus unnecessarily switch to using a conventional ablation modality. Although pacing maneuvers to discriminate the source of a signal are not unique to the PVAC, this device will conceptually record more far-field signals than conventional circular mapping catheters because it has larger electrodes (3 mm vs. 1 mm [Duytschaever et al 2009; *see Recommended Reading*]). Therefore, precise identification of the origin of residual activity, indicated by the electrogram and its relative location and activation when recorded using the PVAC, is crucial to achieving complete PV isolation and relevant to decreasing potential complications and procedure time.

A primary method for determining the origin of electrogram signals on the PVAC is to move the catheter to different positions for mapping as indicated in **Chapters 3** and **4**. Another method is to perform pacing with the PVAC as outlined in **Chapter 7**. This chapter refers to differential pacing with the PVAC used as a mapping catheter in a specific position as directed by the relevant electrogram, and a second pacing catheter maneuvered to different positions.

To Ablate, or Not to Ablate? That is the Question.
The Answer can be Found by Differential Pacing

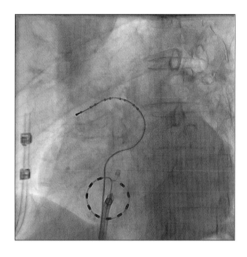

How can electrical signals recorded using the PVAC be differentiated with one additional catheter? This chapter describes the strategy of differential pacing.

The concept of differential pacing is that a far-field signal originating from a specific region, eg, the left atrial appendage (LAA), and recorded on the electrogram of the PVAC, would occur simultaneously or be "pulled in" very near to the pacing stimulus when the pacing catheter is positioned at the specific region of origin of that far-field signal, ie, the LAA. Conversely, if the signal has a true PV origin together with an atrial signal, stimulating the atrium will pull in the atrial far-field signal and "split out" the PV signal. It should be noted that pacing may be necessary not only from the coronary sinus (CS) but also from the LA or the right atrium (RA). Anterior and posterior pacing may be necessary to fully discern the origin of the signal of interest in the anteroposterior direction.

The principle of differential pacing around the PV is described in this chapter with examples that include electrogram tracings and corresponding fluoroscopic views in left anterior oblique (LAO) and right anterior oblique (RAO) projections.

In conventional PV isolation, two catheters—a circular mapping catheter and an ablation catheter—are usually advanced into the LA. The ablation catheter can be utilized for differential pacing. When performing PV isolation with the PVAC, there is usually no second catheter in the LA. This chapter illustrates how all pacing maneuvers are performed adequately with just one steerable CS catheter in addition to the PVAC. Furthermore, transseptal crossing with a steerable CS catheter is demonstrated without the use of a second long sheath or the need for a second transseptal puncture. Of course, differential pacing maneuvers become much easier when multiple catheters are used at different locations simultaneously.

Rationale and Concept of Differential Pacing With the PVAC

The aim of differential pacing is to identify the origin of a given electrogram signal when using a mapping catheter. The mapping catheter, in this case the PVAC, remains in a static position so that the identical signal can be tracked during pacing maneuvers.

The source and direction of the electrical activation wave front defines the delay between electrode signals on a mapping catheter such as the PVAC. During sinus rhythm, the activation wave front reaches the left PVs and the LAA almost simultaneously. Thus, there is usually no delay observed between the signals from these structures (**Figure 1a**).

In contrast, during pacing from the CS the activation wave front usually reaches the LAA before the PV. Therefore, the LAA signal is pulled in and the PV signal is split out in comparison with sinus rhythm signals (**Figure 1b**). However, the delay between the signals varies according to the extent and conduction of muscular connections between the CS and the LA. Differences in anatomy also play a role, which means that the delays shown for the left superior pulmonary vein (LSPV) in this example may not be the case for the left inferior pulmonary vein (LIPV) if the distance to the CS is the same as that from the LAA (**Figure 1b**). In addition, intra-atrial conduction periods can be prolonged, particularly in those patients receiving antiarrhythmic medication. This can lead to delayed atrial signals that mimic a PV origin. In such circumstances, it is mandatory to identify the exact source of the signal on the electrogram in order to confirm that isolation of the PV has been achieved and thus avoid unnecessary RF energy delivery.

Figure 1. (a) Activation during sinus rhythm, and (b) CS pacing.

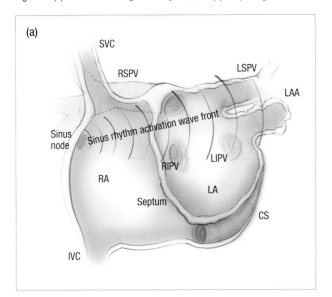

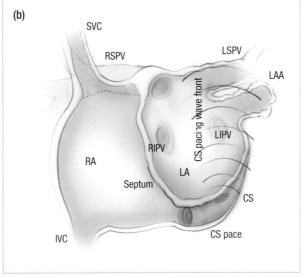

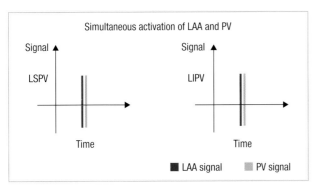

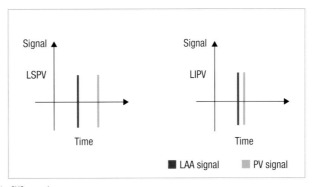

IVC: inferior vena cava; RIPV: right inferior pulmonary vein; RSPV: right superior pulmonary vein; SVC: superior vena cava.

A pacing location inside the LAA (**Figure 1c**) will pull in a far-field signal from the LAA (simultaneously or very shortly after the pacing signal) and split out a PV potential. This location is, therefore, ideal for discerning far-field potentials on the anterior circumference of the PVAC. However, in patients with prolonged intra-atrial conduction times, a far-field atrial signal from the posterior wall can be split out during pacing of the LAA (**Figure 1d**). Thus, it may be necessary to move the pacing catheter to a posterior wall position to confirm complete PV isolation (**Figure 1c**). This position should be far from the PVAC to ensure an absence

of gap pacing, meaning direct capture of the gap that was created from previous ablation using the PVAC. It should be noted that true PV potentials always show a relatively long delay compared with intra-atrial conduction times when pacing outside the PV. This corresponds to the relatively long delays in the opposite direction emanating from the PV, as illustrated with PV pacing in **Chapter 7**. In dubious cases, when interpretation of a delay between two signals is unclear, pacing from the PVAC can provide additional information.

Figure 1. (c) LAA pacing. By pacing the LAA a far-field signal from the LAA is pulled in or is almost simultaneous with the pacing artifact, whereas a signal originating from the LSPV or LIPV is split out. (d) LA anteroposterior delay. When pacing anteriorly in the LAA, the spatial distance to the posterior electrodes of the PVAC can be substantial. This means that a far-field signal originating from the posterior atrium may lead to a considerable delay and be misinterpreted as a real PV signal. Pacing in the posterior LA is advisable in this situation. (e) The final step is stimulation at the posterior wall to confirm complete PV isolation, as shown here in the LSPV, or to reveal true PV signals, as shown in the LIPV.

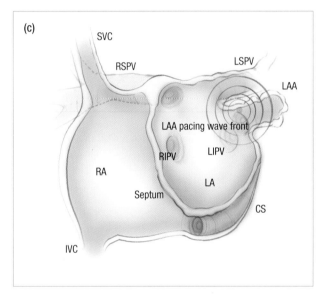
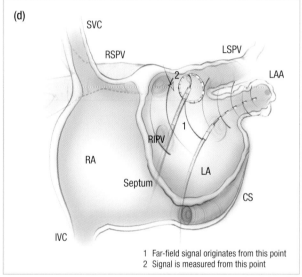
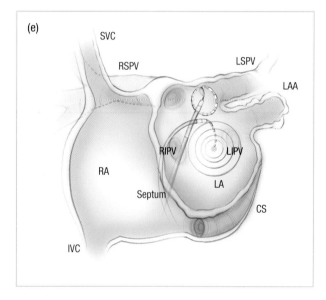

1 Far-field signal originates from this point
2 Signal is measured from this point

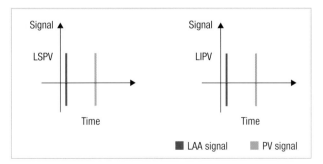
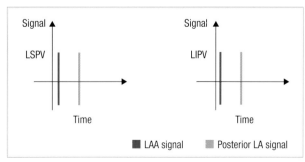
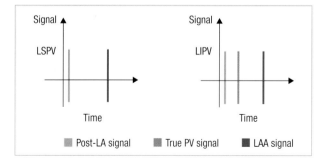

RIPV: right inferior pulmonary vein; RSPV: right superior pulmonary vein; SVC: superior vena cava.

117

Advancing a Coronary Sinus Catheter into the Left Atrium Over the Single Transseptal Puncture Site Without Help from a Second Long Sheath

The PVAC is positioned with a long transseptal sheath into the LA. In most cases, advancing a second pacing catheter (ie, the CS catheter) into the LA is possible without the aid of a second transseptal sheath. If the sheath diameter of the PVAC is significantly larger than the shaft diameter of the PVAC (9.5 F), as is the case with a steerable sheath, then this difference in diameter allows direct passage of the CS catheter into the LA (sometimes called "passive transseptal"). First, the transseptal sheath is pulled back into the RA, then the shaft of the PVAC serves as a guide for advancing the CS catheter into the LA. This approach can be facilitated by utilizing a 4 F CS catheter.

Figure 2a shows the fluoroscopy in the anteroposterior projection, with the PVAC in the LA and a steerable CS catheter *in situ* pulled back from the CS position and tilted upwards to the transseptal puncture site with a clockwise rotation. The tip points towards the puncture site but the aperture seems to be too small to allow entry of a second catheter. This is illustrated by the CS catheter, which flexes to form a curve when pushed forward.

If the difference in diameter between the PVAC shaft and the aperture of the transseptal puncture does not permit direct insertion of the CS catheter into the LA, then the PVAC needs to be withdrawn into the sheath and both catheter and sheath pulled back into the RA (**Figure 2b**). In such circumstances, the central guidewire can be utilized to mark the location of the transseptal puncture site. The CS catheter can then be advanced easily through the puncture site without bending it or needing to apply pressure.

The CS catheter is advanced fully into the LA. Readvancing the sheath with the PVAC over the guidewire into the LA can be challenging because of the jump in diameter between the guidewire (0.032 inch) and the PVAC sheath (**Figure 2c**). This can be overcome by advancing the tip of the PVAC out of the sheath (**Figure 2d**).

Figure 2. (a) Directly advancing the CS catheter into the LA along the PVAC after pulling back the PVAC sheath. The PVAC is shown in the LA ($\downarrow^1$), the CS catheter is pushed towards the septum ($\downarrow^2$), and the sheath is back in the RA (inferior vena cava; $\downarrow^3$). (b) Insertion of the CS catheter into the LA along the PVAC guidewire. The PVAC is shown being withdrawn into the sheath ($\leftarrow^4$), the CS catheter crosses the transseptal puncture site ($\leftarrow^5$), and the PVAC guidewire is situated in the LA ($\leftarrow^6$). (c,d) Readvancing the PVAC sheath into the LA. The PVAC is withdrawn into the sheath ($^7\rightarrow$) with the tip protruding out of it ($^8\rightarrow$) in order to overcome the jump in diameter between the guidewire and the sheath.

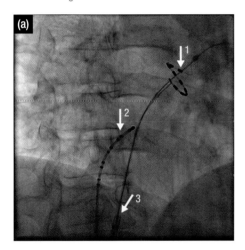 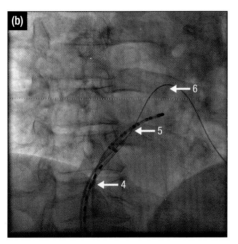 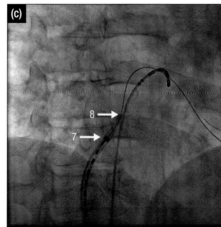 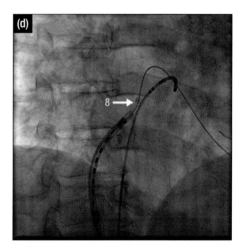

Teaching Case 1: From the Left Superior Pulmonary Vein, Coronary Sinus Pacing

In this chapter a number of teaching cases will be presented, each referring to a slightly different scenario within the same patient and the same PVAC position.

The first case shows a classical example of differential pacing that demonstrates the usefulness of advancing the pacing catheter to the region of interest in order to increase electrical delays between the LAA and the left-sided PVs (**Figure 3**).

The last beat ($\downarrow^1$) of the tracing shows a signal on all PVAC electrodes, which occurs almost simultaneously with CS activation ($\downarrow^1$; *see also* **Figure 1a**). During pacing in the CS, the signal splits out with a narrow gap ($\downarrow^2$; *see also* **Figure 1b**). However, it remains unclear as to whether or not this signal is a PV signal or an atrial signal. Therefore, an additional differential pacing maneuver in the LA is necessary.

Figure 3. (a) Teaching case 1 of CS pacing in the LSPV where the PVAC is situated in the LSPV and the reference catheter is in the CS. (b) Fluorograms, and (c) venograms in LAO and RAO views.

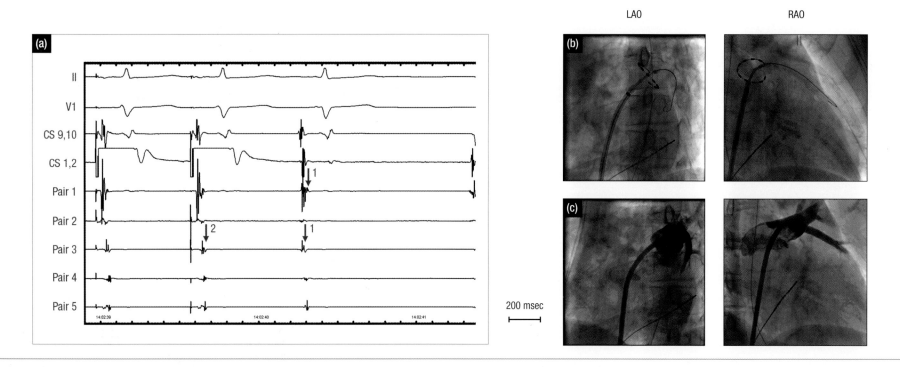

Teaching Case 1: Left Superior Pulmonary Vein With Left Atrial Appendage Pacing

In the same case for the LSPV where the PVAC is situated in an identical position (*see also* **Figure 3**), it is apparent with pacing from the LAA that two signals are present: one is far field from the atrium and pulled in near to the pacing artifact ($\downarrow^1$), while a second signal that emanates from the PV is split out ($\downarrow^2$; **Figure 4**; *see also* **Figure 1c**).

Thus, differential pacing from the LAA is effective in separating overlying signals from the LAA and PV, which occurred simultaneously during sinus rhythm ($\downarrow^3$) and during CS pacing (*see* **Figure 3**).

Figure 4. (a) Teaching case 1 of the LSPV with LAA pacing. (b) Fluorograms, and (c) venograms in LAO and RAO views.

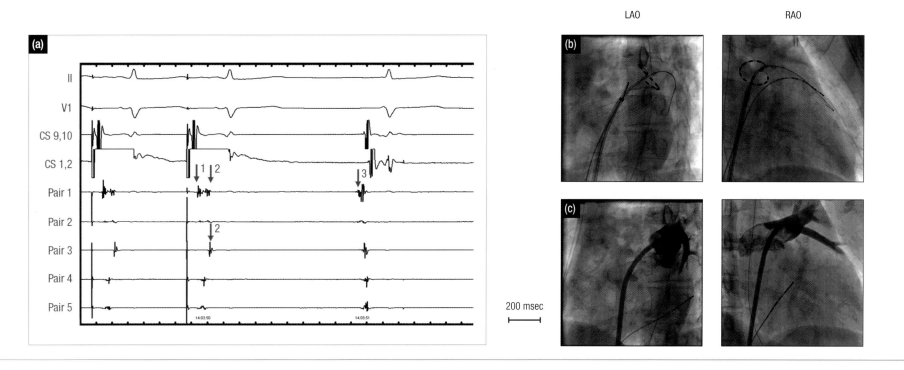

Teaching Case 2: Another Example of Differential Pacing for the Left Superior Pulmonary Vein

Small signals during sinus rhythm (last beat, ↓¹) should always be viewed with caution for PV signals, particularly when they occur simultaneously with atrial signals (↓²; **Figure 5**). If CS pacing is not diagnostic then pacing from the LAA can differentiate between the two signals. During LAA pacing (first two beats), it becomes clear that the large signal is an atrial far-field signal (↓³), whereas the delayed signals are PV signals (↓⁴).

Figure 5. (a) Teaching case 2 shows differential pacing for the LSPV. During sinus rhythm (last beat) the electrogram shows that there is a large signal on electrode 3 of the PVAC (↓²) and smaller signals at the other electrodes (↓¹). It remains unclear which signal originates from the LA and which is from the PV. During pacing from the LAA, the large signal (↓³) is advanced whereas the small signal is split out (↓⁴). This means that the large signal is a far-field LAA signal and the small signals are of PV origin. Therefore, during RF energy delivery the abatement of the small signal is expected but the large signal will persist. (b) Fluorograms, and (c) venograms in LAO and RAO views.

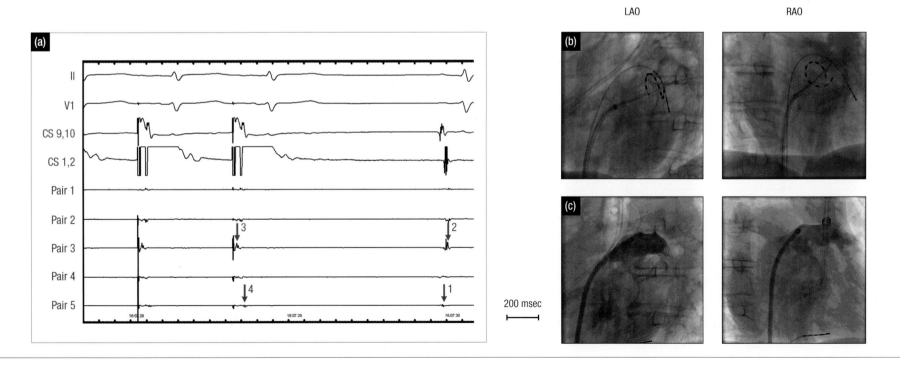

Teaching Case 3: From the Left Inferior Pulmonary Vein, PVAC Position 1, Coronary Sinus Pacing

The concept of differential pacing can be illustrated in the LIPV by using a series of electrograms that confirm the position of the PVAC as remaining static during sinus rhythm, CS pacing, LAA pacing, and posterior left atrial pacing (each pacing maneuver is represented by a schematic in **Figure 1**).

Both a PV signal and an atrial far-field signal could possibly be indicated by the signals shown in **Figure 6a**. During sinus rhythm, a signal is visible on PVAC electrode pairs 1–3 ($\downarrow^1$), which occurs simultaneously with the signal in the CS. During CS pacing (first beat), the signal is delayed after the pacing stimulus ($\downarrow^2$). The exact origin (far-field atrial signal, ie, from the LAA vs. PV signal) remains unclear (*see also* **Figure 1a** and **b**). **Figure 6b** shows the LAO and RAO views of the PVAC positioned in the LIPV and the CS catheter in its standard position within the CS.

Figure 6. (a) Teaching case 3 from the LIPV, PVAC position 1, CS pacing. (b) Fluorograms, and (c) venograms in LAO and RAO views.

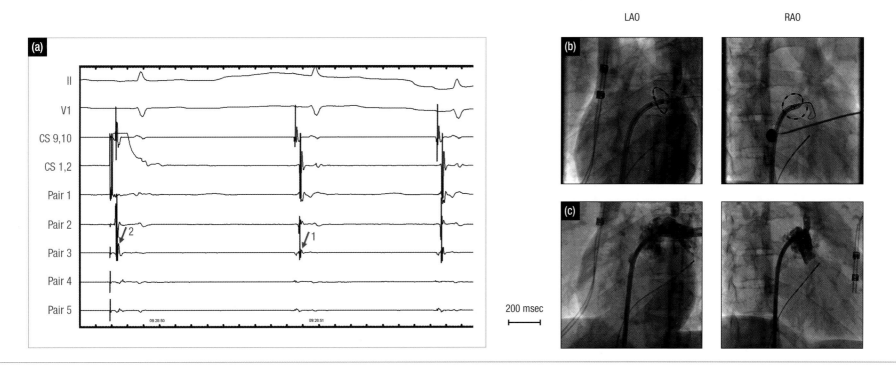

Teaching Case 3: PVAC Position 1, Left Atrial Appendage Pacing

The PVAC is in the LIPV at an identical position to that shown in **Figure 6**. To rule out an LAA far-field signal on using the PVAC, the CS catheter is moved from the CS to the LAA (*see* **Figure 1c**). When pacing from the distal part of the reference catheter in the LAA, the signal on electrode pairs 1 and 2 of the PVAC ($\downarrow^1$) is split out as the delay on the PVAC becomes more prominent, thereby ruling out a far-field signal from the LAA. This suggests a PV signal. However, probatory delivery of RF energy will not result in abolition of the signal in this case. Repeated and extensive RF energy applications without signal abatement would give the operator the illusion that the duty-cycled RF ablation was not effective. The PVAC would also be in undesirable proximity to the posterior wall and the esophagus as a consequence of the posterior location of electrode pairs 1 and 2. Note that the pacing position in the LAA is in the anterior part of the LA, whereas the signal appears at PVAC electrode pairs 1 and 2, which is at the 11 o'clock position posteriorly as observed in the LAO view in **Figure 7b** (*see also* **Figure 1d**). Therefore, an additional differential pacing maneuver is recommended to provide confidence on the source of this signal.

Figure 7. (a) Teaching case 3, PVAC position 1, LAA pacing. (b) Fluorograms, and (c) venograms in LAO and RAO views.

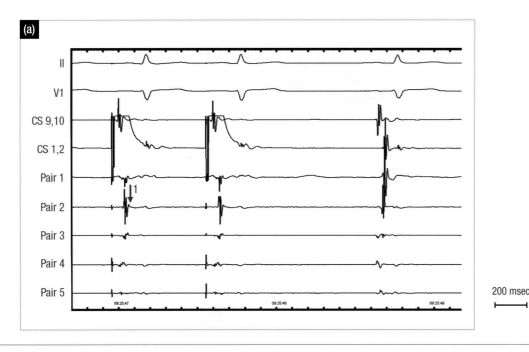

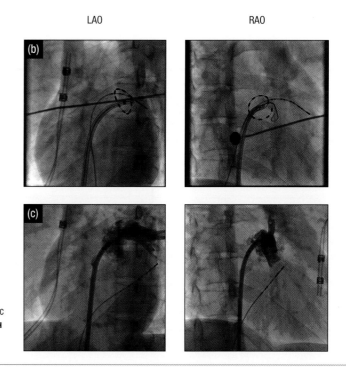

Teaching Case 3: PVAC Position 1, Posterior Left Atrial Pacing

Again, with the PVAC at an identical position in the LIPV to that shown in **Figure 6**, the reference catheter is now withdrawn from the LAA and turned clockwise towards the posterior wall (*see also* **Figure 1e**). When pacing again from the distal pair of the CS reference catheter, which is about 1–2 cm infero-posterior to the PVAC, the signal in question on electrode pairs 1 and 2 of the PVAC occurs simultaneously with the pacing artifact ($\downarrow^1$; **Figure 8a**). Thus, the signal results from a far-field signal of the posterior LA. The pacing occurs at least 1–2 cm distant from the PVAC to avoid gap pacing (*see* **Figure 1e**). Retrospectively, the delay observed during CS pacing in **Figure 6** corresponds to the conduction period between the CS and the posterior LA. As a consequence, this signal is not ablated. If the signals were examined only during CS and LAA pacing (**Figures 6** and **7**) this may have led to their misinterpretation as PV signals. In such circumstances, RF energy delivery would not only be ineffective but potentially harmful in the posterior LA.

Figure 8. (a) Teaching case 3, PVAC position 1, posterior LA pacing. (b) Fluorograms [($\uparrow^2$) pacing site, ($\downarrow^3$) recording site], and (c) venograms in LAO and RAO views.

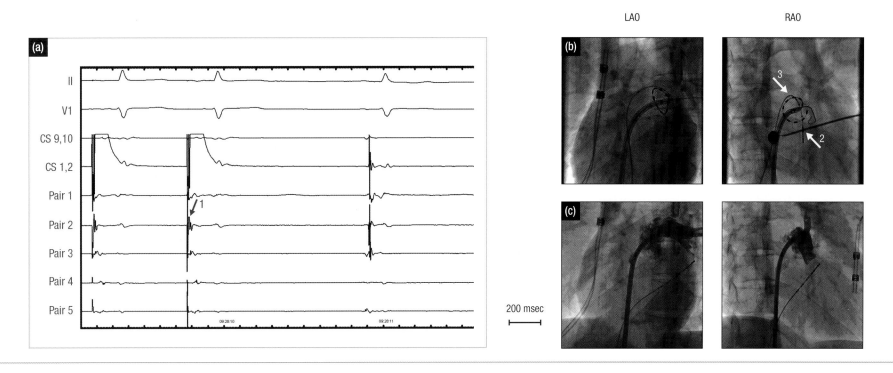

Teaching Case 3: From the Left Inferior Pulmonary Vein, PVAC Position 2

Figure 9 is a second example from the LIPV of the same patient, which demonstrates the value of differential pacing in pulling out real PV signals. The position of the PVAC differs slightly from that seen in position 1 (**Figures 6–8**), as observed on comparison with corresponding PV angiograms. In sinus rhythm (last beat), there is a signal of unclear origin at pairs 1 and 2, as well as at pairs 4 and 5 ($\downarrow^1$) of the PVAC. During CS pacing, a delay after the signal becomes apparent in pairs 1 and 2 ($\downarrow^2$) of the PVAC. However, a delay is also observed on PVAC electrode pairs 4 and 5 ($\downarrow^3$), which means that the origin of the signal on electrode pairs 1 and 2 of the PVAC is not certain (*see also* **Figure 1a** and **b**). Pacing from the CS is, therefore, not diagnostic in this case.

Figure 9. (a) Teaching case 3 from the LIPV, PVAC position 2, CS pacing. (b) Fluorograms, and (c) venograms in LAO and RAO views.

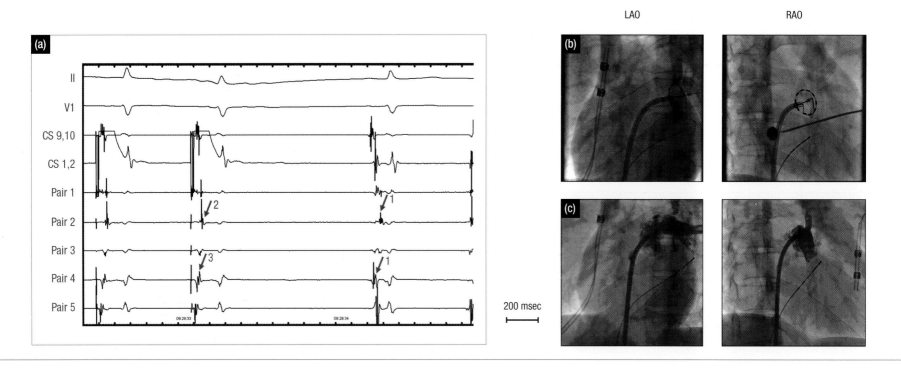

Teaching Case 3: PVAC Position 2, Left Atrial Appendage Pacing

The PVAC is in the LIPV at position 2, which is identical to that shown in **Figure 9**. In order to rule out a far-field signal from the LAA, the reference pacing catheter (CS catheter) is advanced into the LAA (**Figure 10**). Pacing from the distal CS electrode at the tip of the LAA shows an increased delay at electrode pairs 1 and 2 ($\downarrow^1$), thereby ruling out a left atrial far-field signal from the LAA (*see also* **Figure 1c**). The delay at PVAC electrode pairs 4 and 5 is close to the pacing artifact ($\downarrow^2$) and is probably a far-field signal from the atrium.

Figure 10. (a) Teaching case 3, PVAC position 2, LAA pacing. (b) Fluorograms, and (c) venograms in LAO and RAO views.

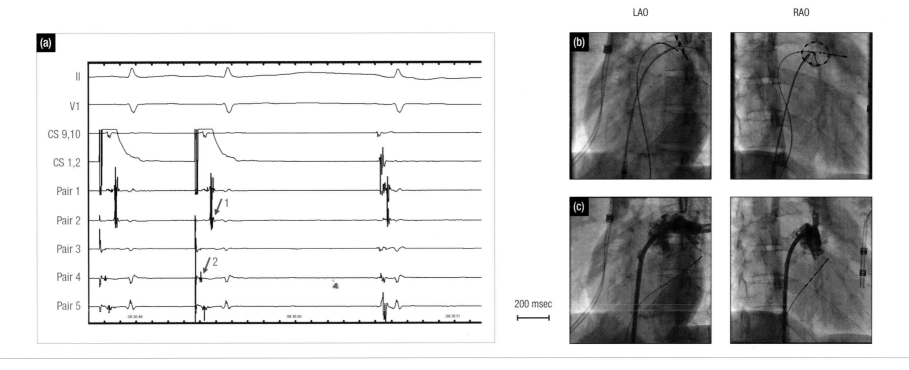

Teaching Case 3: From the Left Inferior Pulmonary Vein, PVAC Position 2, Posterior Left Atrial Pacing

Figure 11 shows the reference catheter in the posterior LA and the PVAC in position 2 in the LIPV (identical case to that shown in **Figure 9**; *see also* **Figure 1e**). The first signal ($\downarrow^1$) of the PVAC signal during sinus rhythm (last beat) occurs simultaneously with the pacing artifact when pacing from the distal pair of the reference catheter. The second part of the PVAC signal is clearly separate ($\downarrow^2$), and therefore rules out a far-field posterior wall signal. It should be noted that the PVAC electrodes of interest (pairs 1–3) are actually directed towards the posterior side. This explains the relatively short interval between the PV signals and the pacing artifact when pacing from the posterior LA ($\downarrow^1$). The signals on PVAC electrode pairs 4 and 5 ($\downarrow^3$) again occur very close after the pacing artifact and are, therefore, far-field signals.

Figure 11. (a) Teaching case 3 from the LIPV, position 2, posterior pacing. (b) Fluorograms [($\uparrow^4$) pacing site, ($\uparrow^5$) recording site], and (c) venograms in LAO and RAO views.

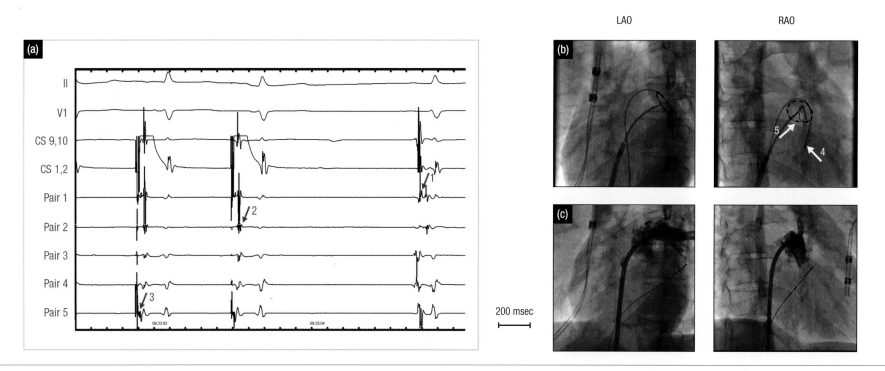

Teaching Case 4: From the Left Inferior Pulmonary Vein, Pacing Distally and Proximally in the Left Atrial Appendage

The CS catheter is placed in the LAA (**Figure 12a**). A large signal is observed on PVAC electrode pairs 3 and 4 ($\downarrow^1$), and a small signal on PVAC pairs 1, 2, and 5 ($\downarrow^2$) during sinus rhythm (first beat) and during pacing from the distal pair of the CS catheter in the LAA (beats 2–5). It is unclear whether these signals are PV signals or far-field signals from the LAA because their timing is simultaneous during sinus rhythm and pacing distally in the LAA.

The proximal CS electrode is located at the base of the LAA, which is much closer to the PV ostium. During pacing from the proximal CS electrode the large signals on electrode pairs 3 and 4 ($\downarrow^3$) are pulled in simultaneously to the pacing signal and are, therefore, far-field signals from the proximal LAA (**Figure 12b**). In contrast, the small signals on PVAC electrode pairs 1, 2, and 5 are split out ($\downarrow^4$). The delay has increased as the site of pacing becomes closer to the site of recording, thereby confirming the origin from within the PV (true PV signals). This again illustrates the principle of differential pacing, namely that when pacing occurs closer to the site of recording, the separation between the signals of interest increases, making diagnosis easier.

Figure 12. (a) Sinus rhythm (first beat) followed by pacing distally in the LAA, and **(b)** pacing the proximal appendage. **(c)** Fluorograms in LAO (top panel) and RAO (bottom panel) views. Pacing is performed either from the distal or proximal pair of the CS catheter; the PVAC is in the LIPV.

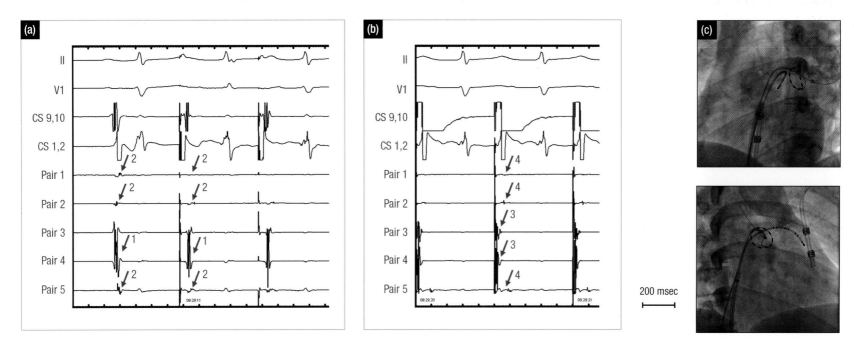

Teaching Case 5: Differential Pacing in the Right Superior Pulmonary Vein

Differential pacing in the right superior pulmonary vein (RSPV) is shown in **Figure 13**. The electrogram shows that there are large signals (↓¹) around the entire circumference of the PVAC during sinus rhythm, and that these signals are not abated despite RF energy delivery. When the pacing electrode is inserted into the LA and pacing is performed from the distal electrode, then all signals are pulled in shortly after the pacing artifact (↓²). Therefore, the signals surrounding the PVAC result from a far-field origin, probably at the left inter-atrial septum. Large far-field signals may be attributed to the relatively large muscle mass of the septum.

Figure 13. (a) Teaching case 5 showing differential pacing in the RSPV: the large signals are the atrial signals (↓²) that occur almost simultaneously with the pacing artefact. (b) Fluorograms showing that the pacing site (³→; LAO) has to be 1–2 cm distant from the PVAC in order to prevent capture of an ablation gap. (c) Venograms in LAO and RAO views.

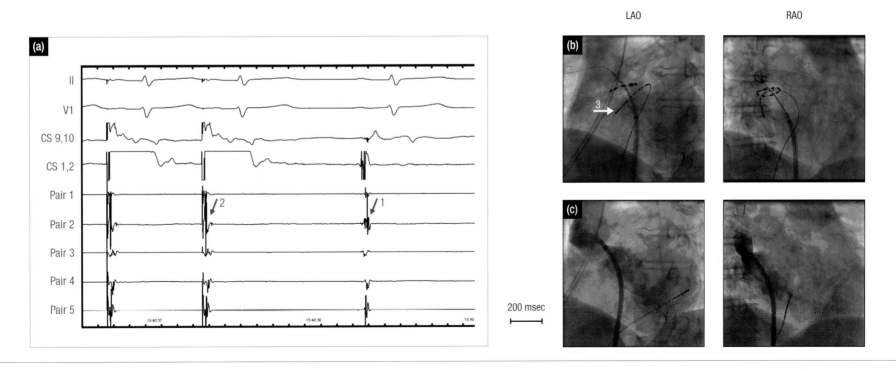

Teaching Case 6: Sinus Rhythm can be Better than Differential Pacing in the Right Superior Pulmonary Vein

This case shows that the RSPV can be well appraised during sinus rhythm and that differential pacing could mask PV potentials (**Figure 14**). Pacing from the LA roof (proximal CS electrode; *see* [↓¹] in the RAO panel of **b**) is less useful than observation during sinus rhythm because the origin of the activation wave front during sinus rhythm is closer to the RSPV. In this example, the gap between the atrial signal (↓²) and PV signal (↓³) is larger during sinus rhythm than during LA roof pacing (↓⁴). Measuring the timing of an RSPV signal in relation to the onset of the P-wave may also help to differentiate the origin of the signal—a signal occurring soon after the onset of the P-wave (within 30 msec) is likely to have an origin in the RA or the superior vena cava (SVC), as described by Shah et al in 2006 (*see Recommended Reading*).

Figure 14. (a) Teaching case 6 showing that pacing of the LA roof from the proximal CS electrode (*see* [↓¹] in the RAO panel of b) is often less useful than observation during sinus rhythm. (b) Fluorograms in LAO and RAO views, and (c) a corresponding LAO venogram.

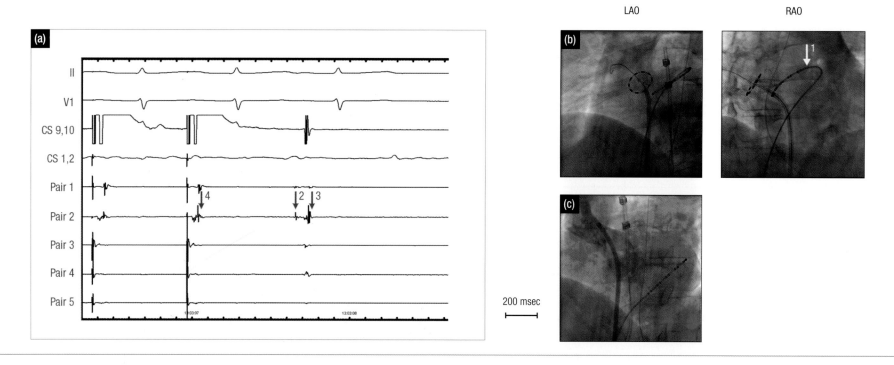

Teaching Case 7: PVAC in the Right Inferior Pulmonary Vein, Pacing in the Coronary Sinus

Figure 15a shows that a signal of unclear origin ($\downarrow^1$) is recorded during sinus rhythm at the right inferior pulmonary vein (RIPV) after initial RF energy applications have been delivered. During CS pacing, the signal becomes smaller and the delay could suggest a PV signal ($\downarrow^2$). The spatial delay between the distal CS electrode (pacing site) and the recording site in the RIPV is, however, considerable.

Figure 15. (a) Teaching case 7: the reference catheter is in the CS and the PVAC is in the RIPV (note the posterior orientation of the guidewire in the LAO view [*see* panel b]). (b) Fluorograms [($\downarrow^3$) pacing site, ($\downarrow^4$) recording site], and (c) venograms in LAO and RAO views.

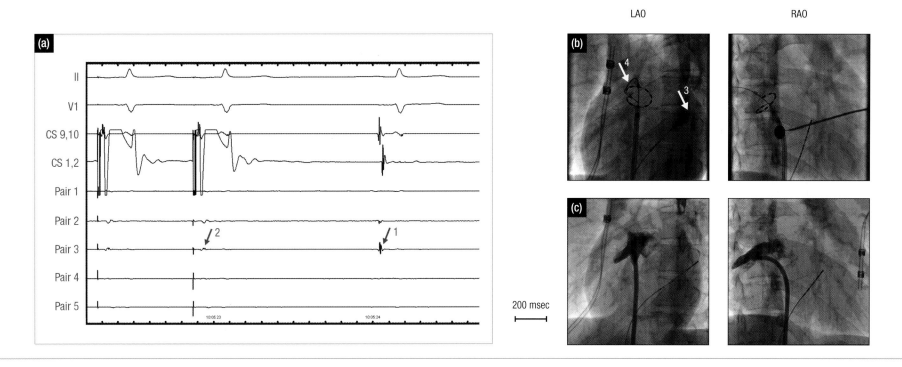

Teaching Case 7: PVAC in the Right Inferior Pulmonary Vein, Pacing in the Right Atrium

Using the same case as that of **Figure 15**, **Figure 16** shows differential pacing in the RA. Far-field signals recorded in right-sided PVs may originate from the RA. Therefore, differential pacing should be performed in the RA when analyzing signals from right-sided PVs. Special consideration should be given to far-field signals from the inter-atrial septum, which can be pulled in or become simultaneous during right atrial septal pacing. Thus, the pacing catheter should be curved towards the right inter-atrial septum as shown in **Figure 16b** where ($\downarrow^1$) is the pacing site.

Figure 16. (a) Teaching case 7 shows that there is a significant delay during right atrial pacing, which makes a far-field right atrial signal unlikely ($\downarrow^2$). However, in this instance delivery of RF energy would not decrease the signal, and can even be harmful as the esophagus may be in the proximity of the posteriorly orientated RIPV (*see also* Figure 2a, Chapter 2). This necessitates a further differential pacing maneuver. The pacing position is located at the right atrial part of the inter-atrial septum. (b) Fluorograms showing the ($\downarrow^1$) pacing site, and (c) venograms in LAO and RAO views.

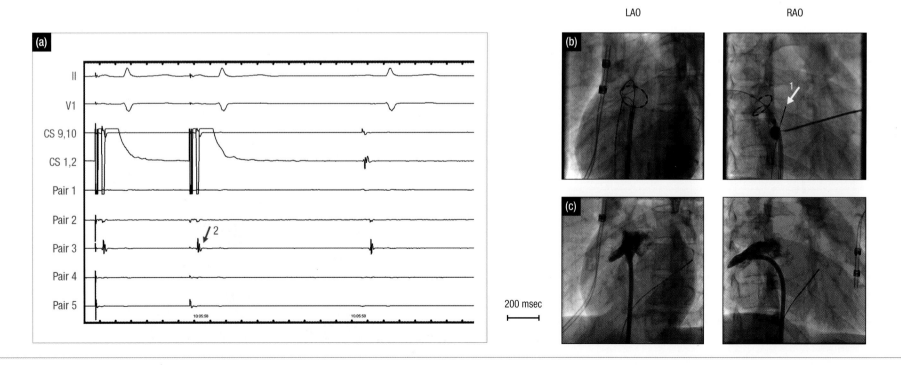

Teaching Case 7: PVAC in the Right Inferior Pulmonary Vein, Pacing in the Posterior Left Atrium

Figure 17 shows that in order to rule out a far-field signal from the LA, the pacing catheter should also be moved to the LA to a pacing position more than 1 cm distal from the PVAC.

Here, a proximal CS electrode is selected for pacing in order to avoid capture of a gap in the previous ablation line and provide true LA pacing (*see* [↓¹]).

Figure 17. (a) Teaching case 7 shows that during LA pacing near the RIPV, from the proximal pair of the CS catheter (CS 9,10; *see* [↓¹] in the RAO panel of b), the signal occurs simultaneously with the pacing artifact (↓²). This indicates that an atrial far-field signal from the upper posterior LA has been recorded—this signal would not decrease even after an extensive RF energy application with the PVAC. (b) Fluorograms, and (c) venograms in LAO and RAO views.

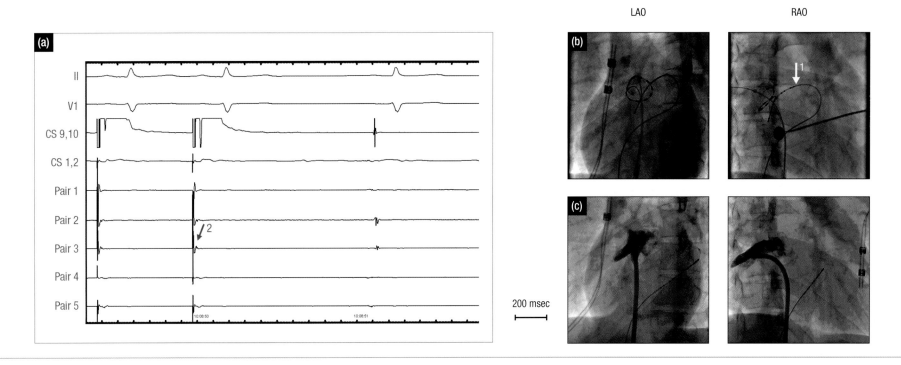

Teaching Case 8: A Second Electrode Position When Pacing Outside of the Right Inferior Pulmonary Vein

This case is an example of RIPV mapping where the reference catheter is pulled back (**Figure 18**). Sometimes it can be difficult to obtain a stable pacing position outside the RIPV. The reference catheter may flip over to the LA roof or to the left side when rotated towards the RIPV, which often sits in a narrow pouch in the right posterior LA region. Therefore, it might be easier to pull the reference catheter back in the transseptal puncture site as shown and pace from the proximal electrode pair.

Figure 18. (a) An example of RIPV mapping where the reference catheter is pulled back and pacing from the proximal pair (*see* [↓¹] in the RAO panel of b) clearly shows the PV origin of this signal (↓²). This can already be observed during sinus rhythm (last beat; ↓³). (b) Fluorograms [(↓¹) pacing site], and (c) venograms in LAO and RAO views.

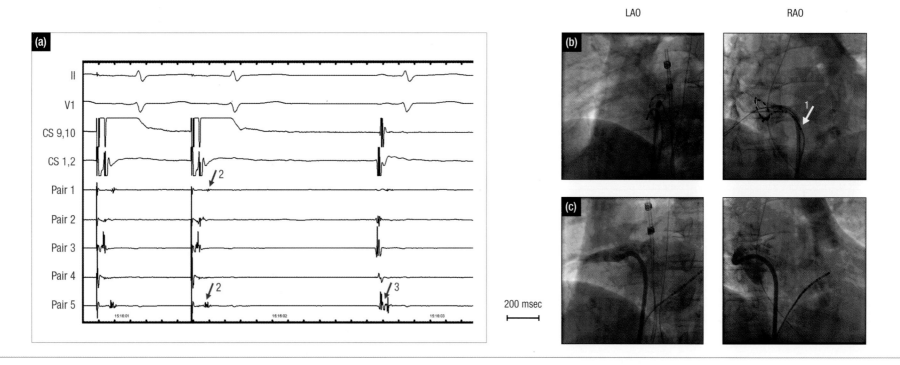

Teaching Case 9: Axial Mapping With the PVAC in a Vein

Unlike a conventional circular mapping catheter, the PVAC has a slide control knob that allows variable elongation and shortening of the shaft axis. Thus, an advantage of the PVAC is that it can be actively elongated for axial mapping, which is especially useful when analyzing the electrical activity going in or out of a vein. This can be illustrated by a case of atrial flutter with a regular atrial activation sequence. In such a scenario, it is clear that the waves of electrical activation move into the vein, in this case the SVC. If the activity emanates from the vein and goes towards the atrium (high to low activation or distal to proximal on the PVAC) this indicates an active SVC. If the activation sequence goes from the atrium up into the vein (low to high activation or proximal to distal on the PVAC) then the SVC is passive with a 1:1 activation ratio. **Figure 19** illustrates a case during atrial flutter in which the SVC is activated passively (proximal to distal activation sequence on the PVAC).

Figure 19. (a) Teaching case 9 shows differential mapping in the SVC. Note that the activation goes from proximal to distal on the PVAC (↑¹), meaning from low to high activation (*see* [↑²] in the RAO panel of b). This indicates that the SVC is activated from the RA and is, therefore, not the active driver of this arrhythmia. (b) Fluorograms in LAO and RAO views.

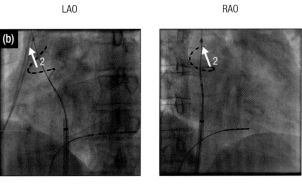

LAO   RAO

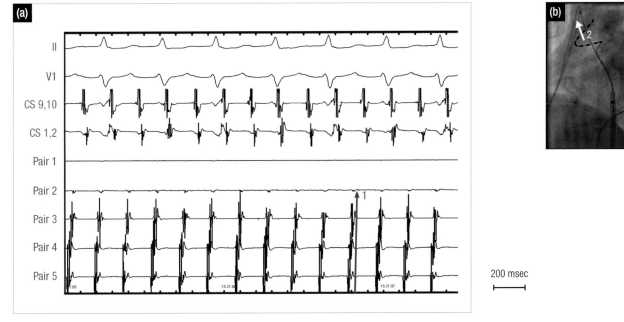

Conclusion

- Correct differentiation between near- and far-field signals on using the PVAC is sometimes needed because the PVAC ablation electrodes have a length of 3 mm, which is comparatively longer than that of conventional circular mapping electrodes (1 mm). Misinterpretation of far-field signals from the RA or the LA for a PV signal may lead to unnecessary RF energy delivery, which may likely be ineffective on signals with far-field origin

- If signal interpretation is unclear during sinus rhythm and pacing from the CS then additional pacing maneuvers from the LA should be performed

- Differential pacing refers to the principle that stimulation near the anatomical origin of a suspected far-field electrogram will pull in the activation sequence of that signal relative to the pacing stimuli, and thus create a timing delay that clearly splits out true PV signals

- Pacing maneuvers can be conducted using a two-catheter technique, eg, PVAC and a steerable CS reference catheter

- Proof of isolation of PVs is a multistep procedure where differential pacing can be an important tool for establishing proof of entrance block

7 | Additional Maneuvers to Ensure Pulmonary Vein Isolation

This chapter describes several additional maneuvers that can be performed to ensure that pulmonary vein isolation has been achieved. One major advantage of the Pulmonary Vein Ablation Catheter (PVAC) is that it allows pacing from each electrode pair. This feature can be used to confirm exit block following initial ablation by pacing from the PVAC after moving it just distal of the ablation line. In addition, pharmacological challenge is another means of confirming that pulmonary vein isolation is achieved. Adenosine plays an important role here: because of its effects on automaticity and conduction, it can help to reveal residual conduction from the pulmonary vein to the left atrium.

Learning Objectives

> To understand the benefit of pacing from each of the electrode pairs of the PVAC after ablation

> To utilize information gained from pacing with the PVAC in conjunction with signal interpretation during sinus rhythm and differential pacing from other catheters

> To realize the limitations of interpretation of the result of pacing if vein capture cannot be confirmed

> To appreciate the value of drug challenges in assessing permanent isolation of the vein

Introduction

Once electrogram analysis during sinus rhythm and pacing suggests that entry block into the pulmonary vein (PV) has been achieved, additional maneuvers are helpful in the confirmation of PV isolation. Differential pacing can be employed to demonstrate entry block (but this requires an additional catheter in the left atrium [LA]), or alternatively the PVAC can be used to demonstrate exit block (from the vein into the LA). One of the advantages of the PVAC is that it can be used to map before the ablation and to deliver radiofrequency (RF) energy, and it can also be used to map and confirm whether or not the ablation has been successful.

In particular, the option to pace from all of the electrode pairs of the PVAC positioned in the vein (ie, distal from the ablation line) can be used to confirm that vein isolation has been achieved. Pacing output is usually set to maximum to ensure capture of the vein muscle, but can be decreased if far-field capture of the atrium is suspected. Finally, temporary vein isolation should be excluded by additional pharmacological tests ("drug challenge"), and non-PV foci should be sought (eg, origin from the superior vena cava [SVC]).

The Concept

Use of pacing from the PVAC after initial energy applications is illustrated in **Figures 1–3**. These show tracings from the PVAC (positioned slightly inside the left superior pulmonary vein [LSPV]) and the coronary sinus (CS) catheter. During sinus rhythm (**Figure 1**), a large double potential is apparent in all of the PVAC recordings (↓). This is almost certainly a PV potential because: (i) the potential is seen in all the PVAC recordings (and not only in the part of the catheter positioned at the anterior ridge between the vein and the left atrial appendage [LAA]), and (ii) the signal timing in respect to the far-field atrial signal and the P-wave suggests a PV potential.

Figure 1. During sinus rhythm a large double potential is apparent in the PVAC recordings.

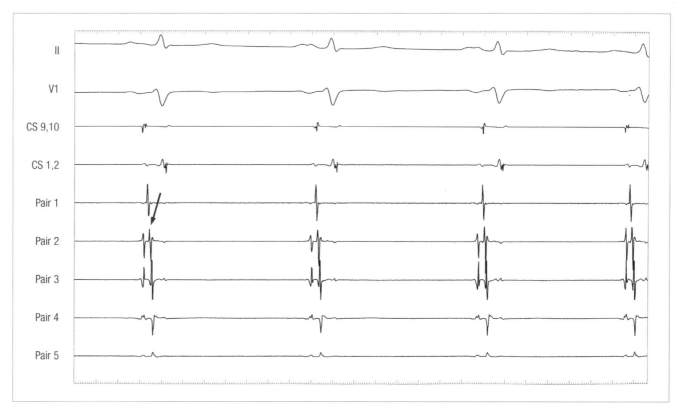

200 msec

During CS pacing (**Figure 2**), the conduction time from the far-field atrial signal to the second potential increases (∗), suggesting that this is indeed a PV potential.

Figure 2. Confirmation of a PV potential during CS pacing.

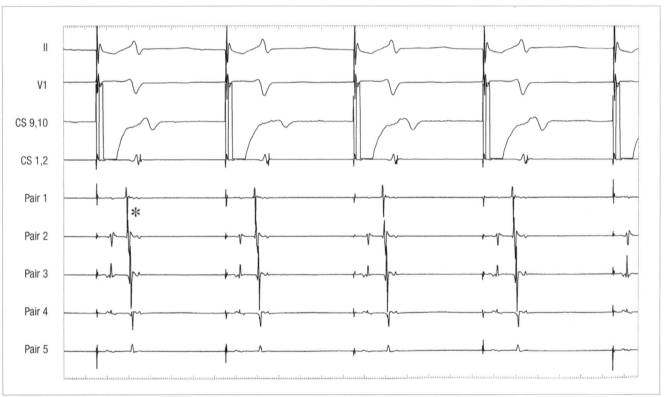

200 msec

Another way to confirm that this is a PV potential is to pace from the PVAC. **Figure 3** shows pacing from PVAC pair 4 with 1:1 conduction into the LA and a long conduction time to the atrium (a far-field signal is observed in both PVAC and CS recordings [↑]) except in beat 3 (∗). During this beat, the pacing stimulus captures both the vein muscle and the LA, which means, therefore, that the conduction time to the atrium is short. It is important to be attentive of the conduction time when a 1:1 PV-LA correlation is observed. If it is short, far-field capture of the LA may be the reason and may require no further ablation. In contrast, when 1:1 conduction is associated with a long conduction time, vein capture and (slow) conduction into the LA via antral tissue may be the cause. In such a situation, additional ablations may be required.

Figure 3. Confirmation of a PV potential by pacing from the PVAC.

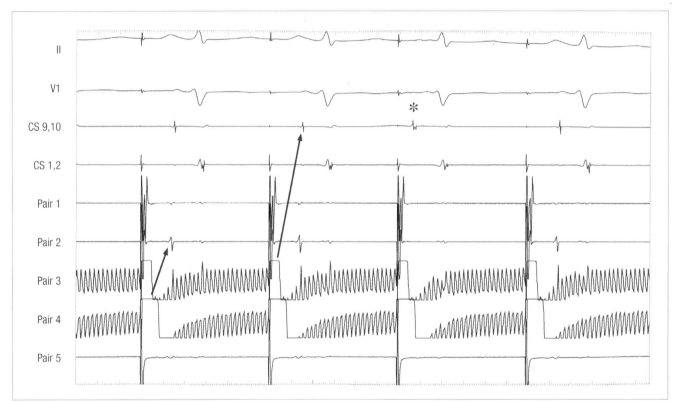

200 msec

Residual Conduction From the Vein into the Left Atrium

Figure 4 shows the recordings from the PVAC while it is positioned in the LSPV following ablation. During pacing from the proximal CS, it is difficult to ascertain whether or not there is a tiny PV potential (↓) in electrode pairs 1 and 5. Entrance block can also be demonstrated by: (i) comparing atrial signals with template signals before ablation, and (ii) pacing of the LAA. If these maneuvers are not possible (eg, atrial fibrillation [AF] at baseline, no second catheter in the LA) then pacing from one of the pairs of the PVAC positioned distal to the ablation line can help to ensure isolation.

Figure 4. Recording from the PVAC when positioned in the LSPV following ablation.

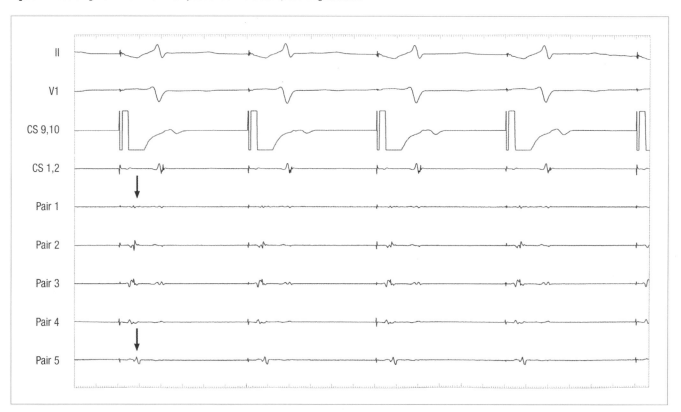

200 msec

Pacing at maximum output from pair 5 shows that the atrial rhythm is dissociated from the paced rhythm (**Figure 5**). However, given the absence of any potential after the pacing signal, it is uncertain as to whether the vein muscle was actually captured. Thus, the pacing does not answer the question of whether the vein is isolated or not (nondecisive). The PV potential can frequently become embedded within the pacing signal; the atrial signal is far-field. In such a case, additional differential pacing maneuvers are required in order to confirm that isolation has been achieved.

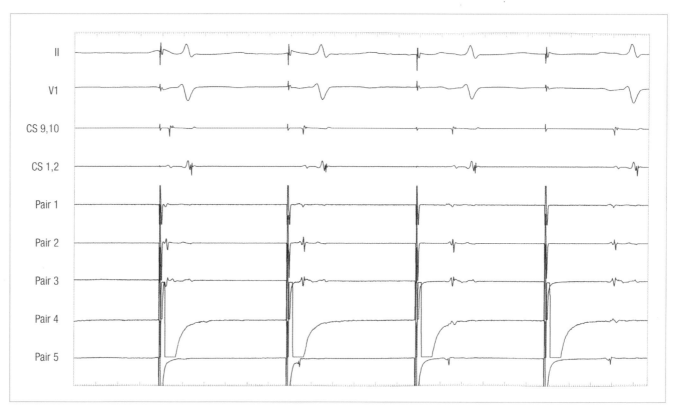

Figure 5. Dissociation of atrial rhythm from the paced rhythm following pacing at maximum output.

200 msec

Stimulation from pair 1 shows that there is a 1:1 correlation between the stimulus and the atrial signal in PVAC and CS recordings (**Figure 6**). The presence of a long (130 msec) stimulus-to-atrium interval (Stim-A interval) in pairs 2–4, which is measured to the atrial signal in the CS recordings, is compatible with PV capture and exit conduction via a gap in the ablation line. Alternatively, far-field capture and direct PV capture with local latency because of a delay within sleeves could also result in a 1:1 correlation with a long Stim-A interval (↓). Additional ablation (ie, from pairs 1 and 5) resulted in complete isolation with demonstration of both entry and exit block. The far-field atrial signal did not change after additional ablation. Note that the CS catheter is relatively far in, and the distal pair shows a ventricular signal.

Figure 6. A 1:1 correlation between the stimulus and the atrial signal in PVAC and CS recordings following stimulation from electrode pair 1.

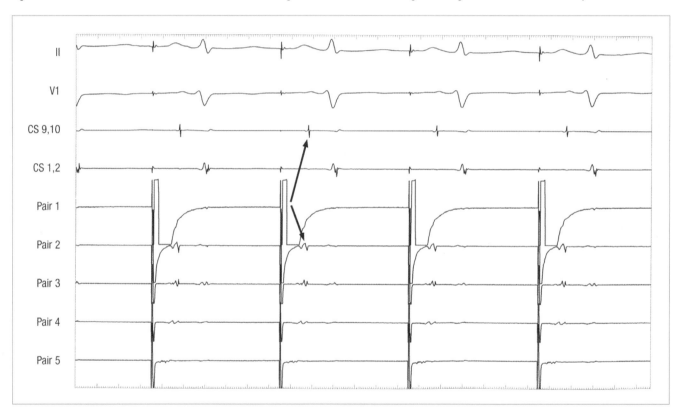

Clear Vein Isolation Demonstrated by Exit Pacing

Following ablation, the PVAC is positioned in the LSPV. During CS pacing (**Figure 7**), a large far-field atrial signal is seen, especially in pairs 2–4, (↓), which is most likely to be a far-field signal from the LAA because of the typical timing of the LAA signal (normally <60–80 msec) and the signal seen in the electrode pairs facing the LAA. Although the electrograms during sinus rhythm and CS pacing would also help to differentiate the origin of this signal, exit pacing is useful to confirm the diagnosis of entrance block and to confirm exit block.

Figure 7. A large far-field atrial signal observed during CS pacing is most likely to be from the LAA.

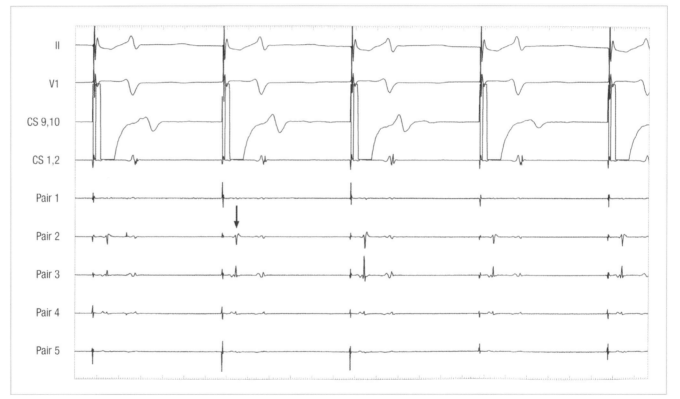

200 msec

Figure 8 shows pacing from pair 4 and capture of the vein muscle as demonstrated by the large signal following the stimulation signal. However, the left atrial signal (∗) is dissociated from the pacing, proving isolation of the vein.

Figure 8. Pacing from pair 4 and capture of the vein muscle as demonstrated by the large signal following the stimulation signal.

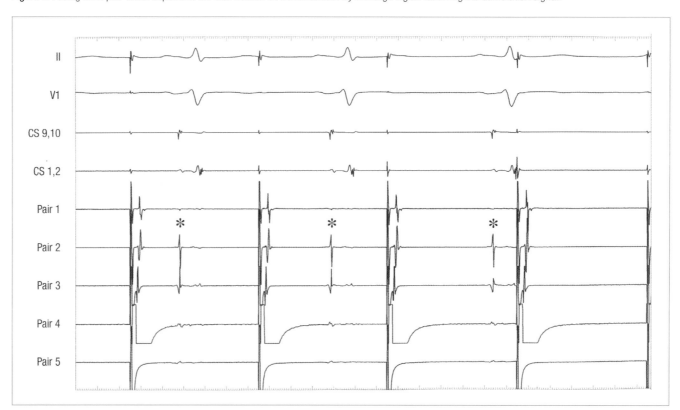

200 msec

Inconclusive Results With Exit Pacing

Following ablation, the PVAC is positioned in the LSPV. During stimulation from pair 3, a 1:1 correlation between the pacing signal and the atrial signal is observed (**Figure 9**). In addition, there is a short Stim-A interval (measured in this case to the atrial signal in the CS recordings [↑] because there is no atrial signal in the PVAC recordings). Thus, exit pacing is nondecisive, which could be a result of either far-field capture of the LA or because the vein has not yet been isolated and conduction out of the vein is still rapid. One option would be to change (decrease) the pacing output to ascertain whether or not this is far-field capture of the atrium.

Figure 9. A 1:1 correlation between the pacing signal and the atrial signal is observed during stimulation from pair 3.

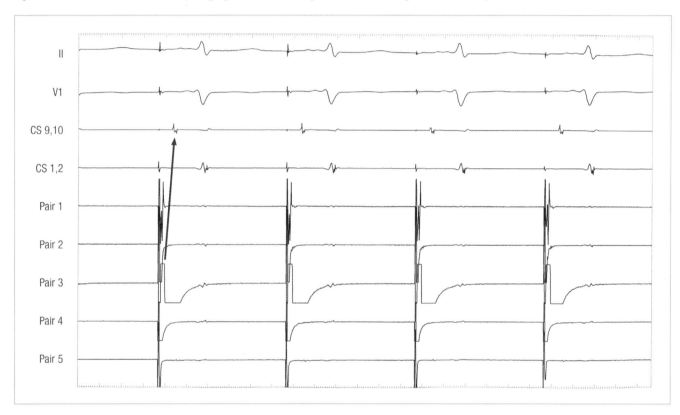

Incomplete Isolation of the Vein

Figure 10 shows a small second potential in pair 4 of the PVAC (↓), which is positioned in the left inferior pulmonary vein (LIPV) after four initial proximal RF energy applications. Here, it is difficult to ascertain whether or not this is still a vein potential requiring additional lesions or a split atrial signal after energy application. This is a very common finding.

Figure 10. Recording showing a small second potential in pair 4 of the PVAC positioned in the LIPV.

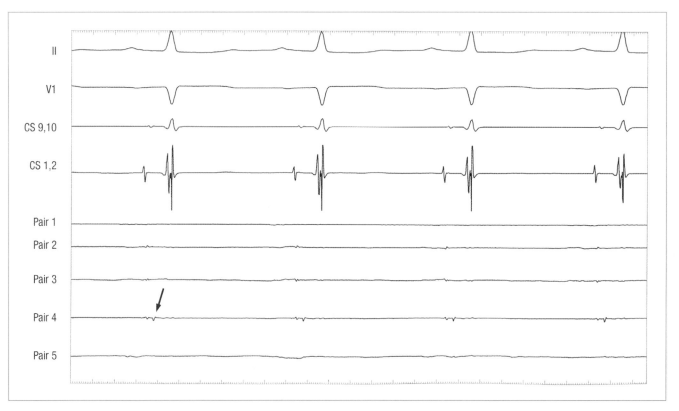

During CS pacing (**Figure 11**), a significantly delayed vein potential becomes visible in pairs 3–5, (↓), and pacing from pair 4 (**Figure 12**) shows 1:1 capture of the atrium and a long conduction time from the stimulus to the atrial signal (↑).

Figure 11. A significantly delayed vein potential becomes visible in pairs 3–5, during CS pacing.

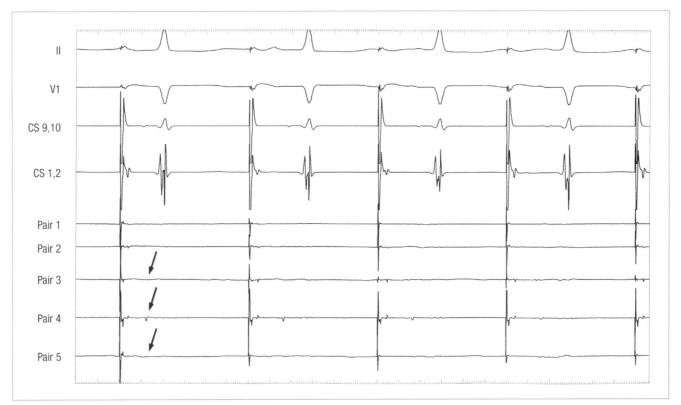

200 msec

Figure 12. Pacing from pair 4 shows 1:1 capture of the atrium and a long conduction time.

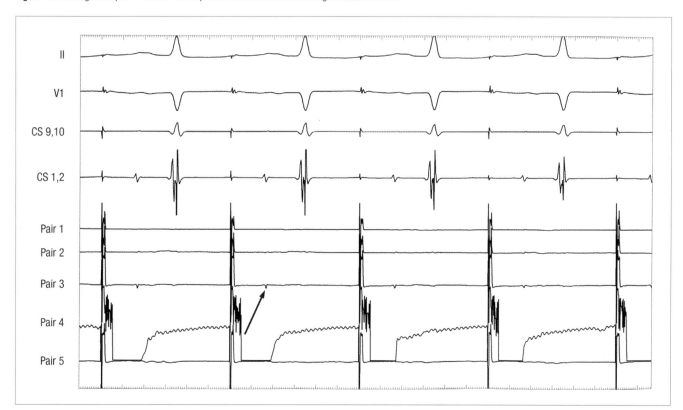

200 msec

Electrograms are Not Decisive for Whether or Not Isolation Has Been Achieved

Figure 13 shows a double potential in pairs 2 and 3 (↓) while the PVAC is positioned in the LIPV after initial ablations. In such a situation, it is difficult to ascertain whether this is due to a residual vein potential or a split atrial signal.

Figure 13. A double potential in pairs 2 and 3 is seen while the PVAC is in the LIPV after initial ablations.

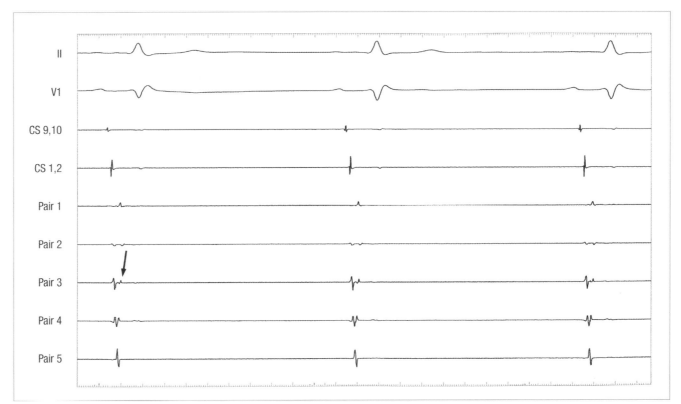

CS pacing delays both signals, and the origin of the second potential remains unclear (**Figure 14**). Although this vein does not seem isolated, based upon the entrance criteria and even with the limited information of these two tracings (sharp potentials, late timing after the P-wave during sinus rhythm, and the fact that a far-field signal is unlikely in the LIPV in all electrodes), exit pacing may confirm that additional lesions are required.

Figure 14. CS pacing delays both signals; the origin of the second potential remains unclear.

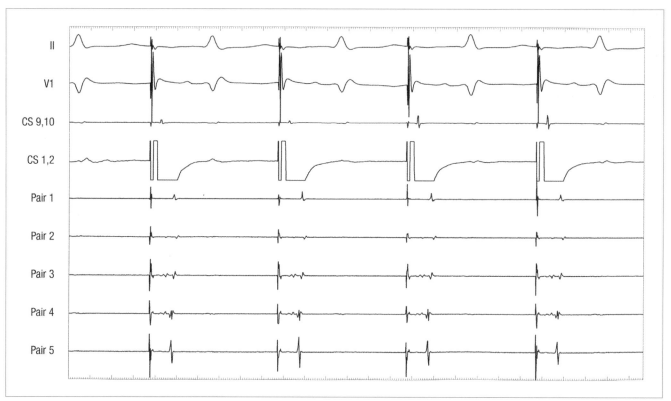

200 msec

Additional Maneuvers to Ensure Pulmonary Vein Isolation

Pacing from pair 2 of the PVAC clearly demonstrates capture of vein muscle and 1:1 conduction into the LA with a long conduction time to the far-field atrial signal (↓), which suggests a gap in the ablation line and the need for additional lesions (**Figure 15**).

Figure 15. Capture of vein muscle and 1:1 conduction into the LA.

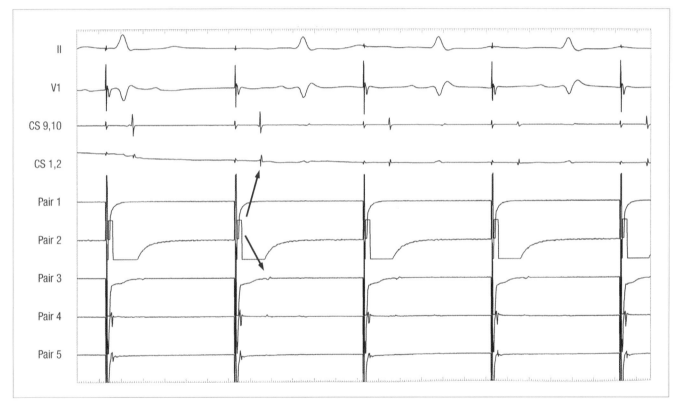

200 msec

Intermittent Residual Conduction From the Vein to the Left Atrium

Figure 16 shows an example of 1:1 capture of the vein muscle (∗) and 2:1 conduction into the LA with a very long delay (↑) during pacing from pair 1, indicating that additional lesions have to be created.

Figure 16. A 1:1 capture of vein muscle and 2:1 conduction into the LA.

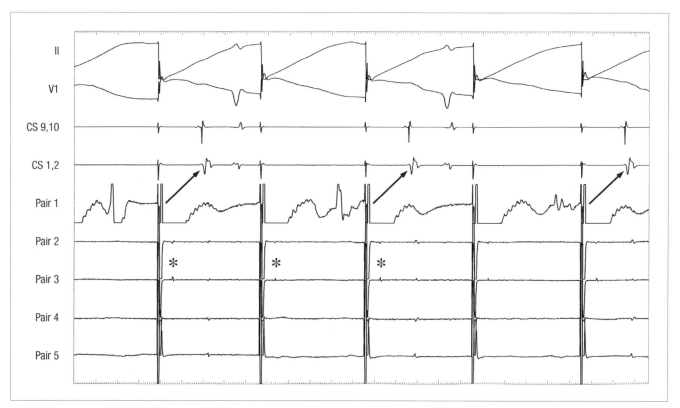

Isolation of the Vein and Uncertain Capture of the Vein Musculature

Figure 17 shows capture of the vein muscle (∗) while the PVAC is positioned in the right superior pulmonary vein (RSPV). However, there is no conduction into the atrium as shown by the dissociated (sinus) rhythm. One caveat is that the post stimulus artifact can sometimes mimic PV capture, especially if the signal is as small as that seen in this example. In contrast, clear capture of the vein can be observed in **Figure 8**.

Figure 17. Capture of the vein muscle while the PVAC is in the RSPV.

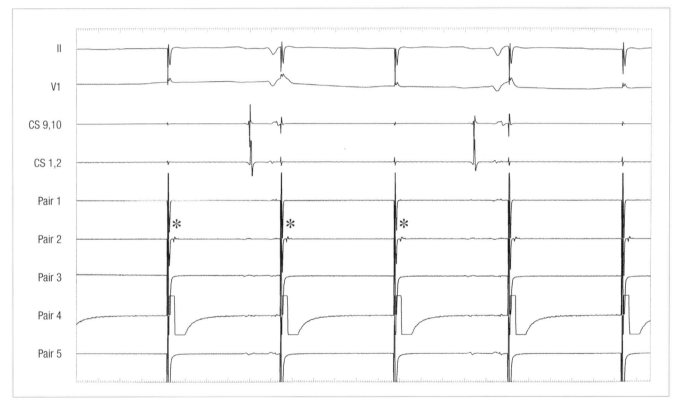

Pharmacological Testing

Use of adenosine, an endogenous nucleoside that exerts its electrophysiological properties mainly by activating a number of outward potassium currents, has been established as one way of determining whether PV isolation is permanent or only temporary. Two main mechanisms for how adenosine restores LA-PV conduction are discussed. Adenosine may either: (i) set off epicardial fibers with a distal insertion, as suggested by the observation that reappearing PV potentials are seen distal within the PV, or (ii) restore excitability of previously thermally injured fibers by hyperpolarizing the cell membrane and reducing action potential duration and refractoriness of cells previously disturbed by the RF energy delivery. In addition, adenosine is also able to influence the electrical activity in the vein.

Reconnection of a previously isolated vein with adenosine

Figure 18 shows reconnection of the right inferior pulmonary vein (RIPV) after intravenous adenosine injection (15 mg). The PVAC is positioned in the vein, and with the third beat the PV potential reappears (↓) and, after a few more seconds, disappears again (∗) (**Figure 19**).

Figure 18. Reconnection of the RIPV after intravenous adenosine injection.

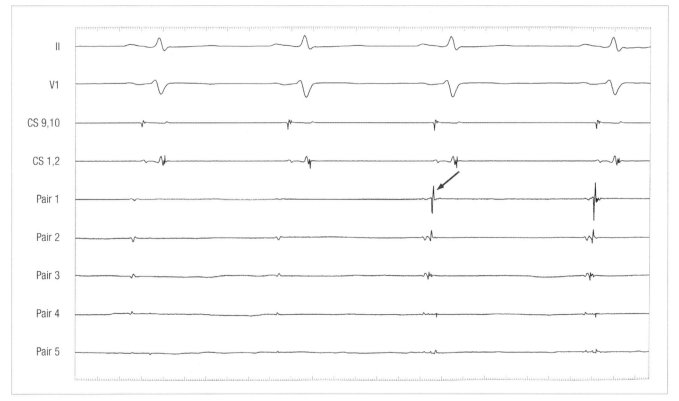

200 msec

Figure 19. Reappearance and disappearance of the PV potential.

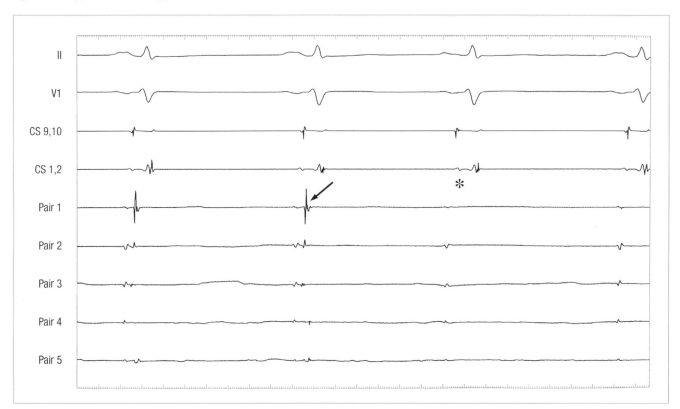

200 msec

No reconnection with adenosine

Figure 20 shows a negative adenosine challenge. Despite atrioventricular (AV) block after adenosine injection there is no reconnection of the LSPV.

Figure 20. A negative adenosine challenge shows that despite AV block after adenosine injection there is no reconnection of the LSPV.

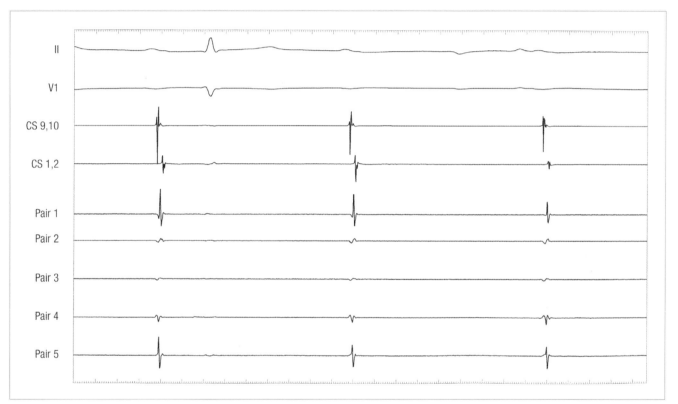

During stimulation from pair 5 of the PVAC (**Figure 21**) there is no conduction into the LA. However, the caveat here is that there is no clear PV potential after the stimulus artefact, and so vein capture is not confirmed.

Figure 21. No conduction into the LA.

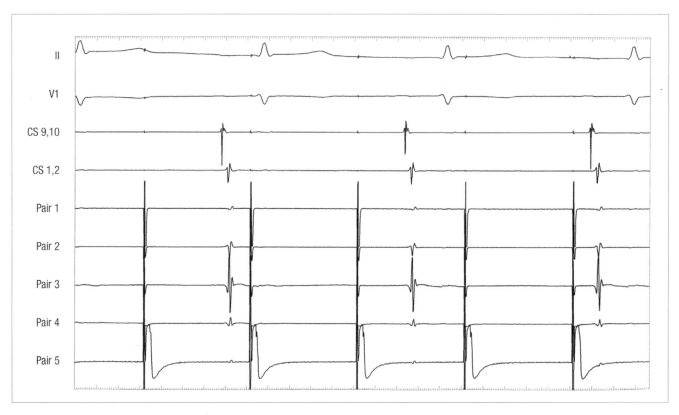

200 msec

Reconnection after adenosine

Figure 22 shows a recording of the PVAC positioned in the LSPV, which had been isolated after ablation. During CS stimulation and after intravenous adenosine injection (15 mg), a small vein potential (↓) reappears with a long conduction time from the far-field atrial signal.

Figure 22. Reappearance of a small vein potential in the isolated LSPV during CS stimulation and after intravenous adenosine injection.

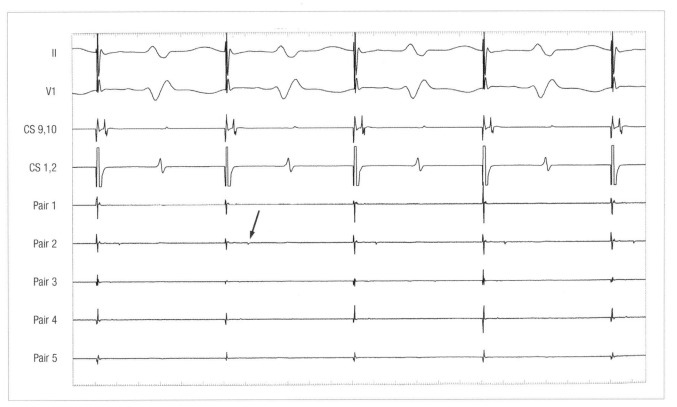

200 msec

Following adenosine injection, pacing from pair 5 (**Figure 23**) results in 1:1 conduction to the LA (↑), again with a long conduction time to the far-field atrial signal (∗). This suggests that isolation of this vein has not been achieved and that additional ablation is needed.

Figure 23. A 1:1 conduction to the LA following adenosine injection suggests that isolation has not been achieved.

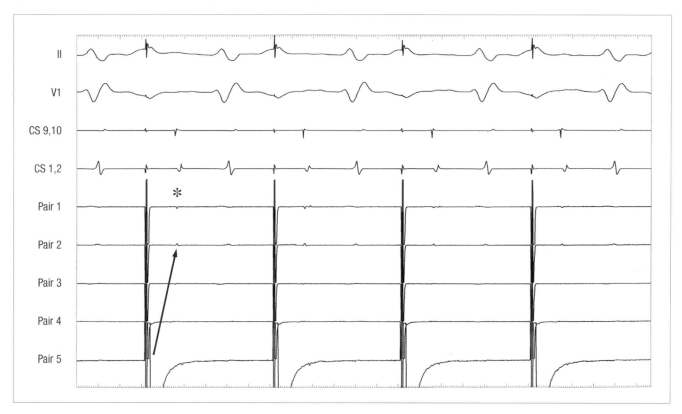

200 msec

Reconnection after adenosine: confirmation by signal interpretation and exit pacing

Figure 24 shows a recording of the PVAC positioned in the LIPV, which had been isolated after ablation and assessed with CS pacing. Pacing from pair 5 of the PVAC positioned inside the vein demonstrates no relation to the atrial signal. However, there is no clear PV potential so vein capture is not confirmed.

Figure 24. Assessment of the isolated LIPV with CS pacing following ablation.

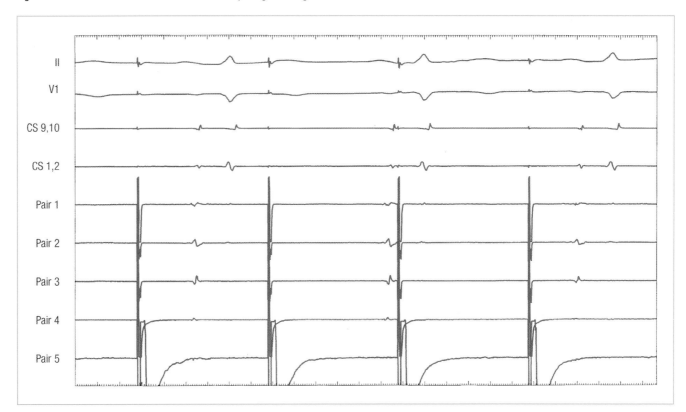

200 msec

Figure 25 shows that, after injection of 6 mg of adenosine, AV block is observed and a large PV potential reappears in the last two atrial beats (∗) during pacing from the CS.

Figure 25. AV block is observed following injection of adenosine.

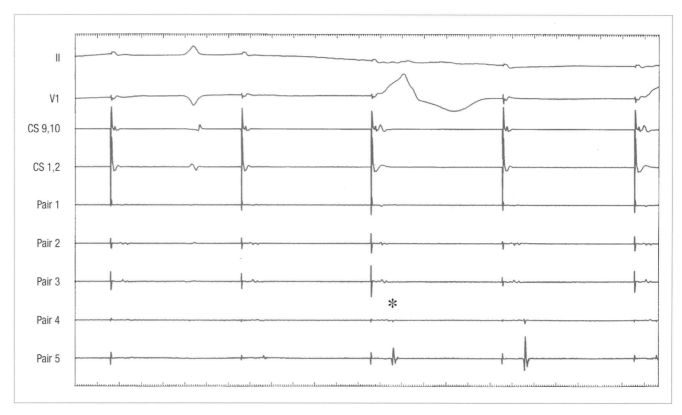

Figure 26 shows that, during the late phase of the adenosine effect, pacing from pair 5 of the PVAC positioned inside the vein demonstrates a 1:1 correlation to the atrial signal. Although there is still no clear PV potential, this observation is suggestive of acute reconnection of the vein with transient exit conduction during pacing. Therefore, additional lesions are needed from the electrode pairs showing the PV potential.

Figure 26. A 1:1 correlation to the atrial signal is suggestive of acute reconnection of the vein with transient exit conduction during pacing.

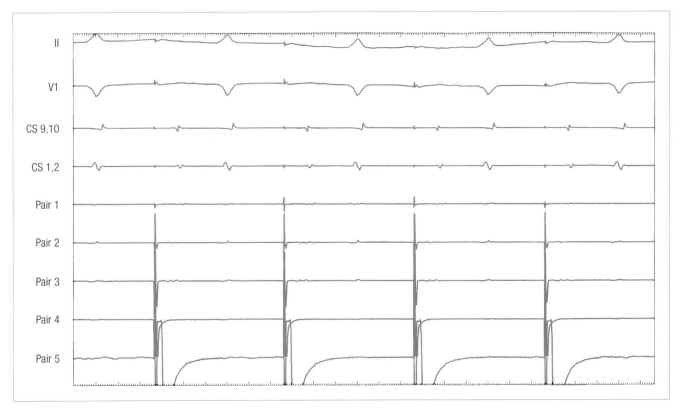

200 msec

Conclusion

- Pacing is utilized to confirm entry block and exit block, and pharmacological testing can help to assess whether or not the goal of the procedure has been achieved. However, it is sometimes difficult to ascertain if there is capture of the vein muscle during stimulation with the PVAC

- **Figure 27** summarizes the different situations encountered during stimulation with the PVAC after initial ablations have been performed. This algorithm is most helpful when a 1:1 correlation between the stimulus and the atrial response is observed together with a long conduction time (*see* **Figures 3**, **6**, and **23**), and in cases where clear capture of the vein is seen and there is no conduction to the atrium (*see* **Figures 8** and **17**)

- The most common situation is uncertain capture of the vein (*see* **Figures 5** and **24**), for which the scenario portrayed in the algorithm is inconclusive. Similarly, when there is a 1:1 correlation between stimulus and atrial response with a short conduction time (*see* **Figure 9**), then again, the scenario in the algorithm is inconclusive. In addition, baseline conduction delay because of the structural changes in the atrium or the effects of the lesions will make the definition of long conduction time difficult

- The effect of antiarrhythmic drugs also needs consideration. Despite these limitations, this algorithm may help in interpreting difficult signals after initial ablation without the need for a second catheter in the LA

Figure 27. Different scenarios encountered during stimulation with the PVAC after initial ablation.

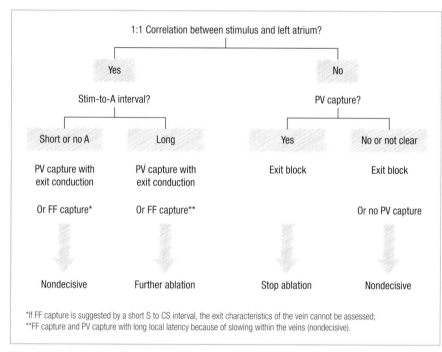

*If FF capture is suggested by a short S to CS interval, the exit characteristics of the vein cannot be assessed;
**FF capture and PV capture with long local latency because of slowing within the veins (nondecisive).

FF: far-field; short S: short sinus; Stim-to-A: stimulus to atrium.

8 | Unusual Tracings During Ablation Using the PVAC

This chapter describes some unusual tracings and observations made during procedures involving the use of the Pulmonary Vein Ablation Catheter (PVAC).

Learning Objectives

> *To appreciate mapping of arrhythmogenic pulmonary veins*

> *To understand mapping of non-pulmonary vein foci*

> *To understand mapping of undirectional left atrial pulmonary vein block*

> *To acknowledge vagal response during ablation*

Mapping of a Triggering Left Superior Pulmonary Vein Using the PVAC

Figure 1a shows that short-coupled ("P on T") ectopy was observed at baseline on mapping within the left superior pulmonary vein (LSPV). During ectopy, an isolated pulmonary vein (PV) signal (↓, pairs 1 and 2) preceded activation of the PV (from pair 5 to pair 1, ↑) and activation of the left atrium (LA) (from the distal coronary sinus [CSD], ie, CS 1,2, to the proximal coronary sinus [CSP], ie, CS 9,10). In **Figure 1b**, after proximal radiofrequency (RF) energy ablation, PVAC mapping within the LSPV revealed that there was an absence of PV potentials and that there was no longer any PV firing.

Electrical isolation was confirmed by mapping with a conventional circular mapping catheter (CMC) (not shown).

Figure 1. Mapping of PV ectopy with the PVAC (a) at baseline in the LSPV, and (b) after proximal ablation.

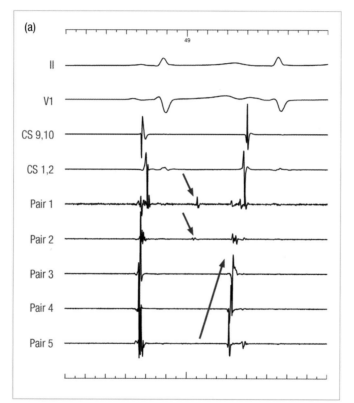
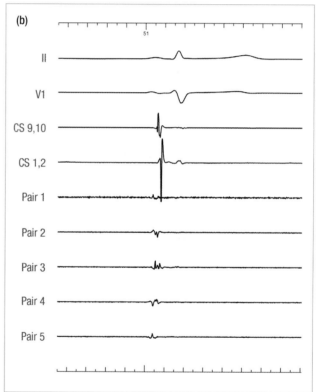

100 msec

Mapping and Ablation of Pulmonary Vein-Mediated Atrial Tachycardia Using the PVAC

On carrying out proximal PVAC mapping (**Figure 2**) there was a repeated initiation of atrial tachycardia (**Figure 3**). During sinus rhythm (beats 1 and 2), clear PV potentials were observed at the LA-PV junction (↓). At the time of the first ectopic beat (beat 3), PV signals (↓, pairs 1 and 2) preceded further activation of PV (from pair 1 to pair 5) and activation of the LA (from CSP to CSD). Furthermore, during subsequent tachycardia beats, the PV potentials at the right superior pulmonary vein (RSPV) (pairs 1 and 2) preceded LA activation (↙, from CSP to CSD).

Figure 2. Mapping of a triggering PV with the PVAC at the ostium of the RSPV.

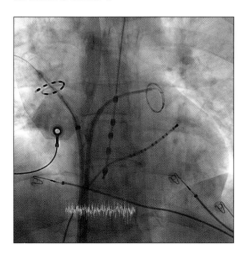

Figure 3. PVAC mapping at the ostium of the RSPV during initiation of atrial tachycardia.

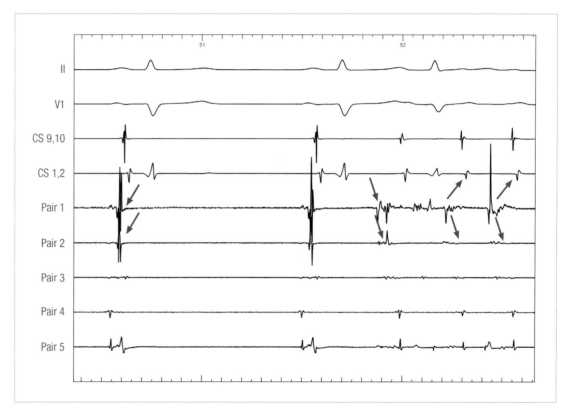

100 msec

In this case (the same as described above), on initiation of RF energy, atrial tachycardia still occurred from within the RSPV (↓; **Figure 4a**). During the first 1 sec of RF energy delivery atrial tachycardia was terminated by ablation.

Immediately after the RF application (**Figure 4b**), PVAC mapping revealed an early signal (before CS potentials and <40 msec from the onset of the P-wave) with a small amplitude (∗), which suggested that these potentials were far field from the superior vena cava (SVC).

Figure 4. Ablation of pulmonary vein tachycardia with the PVAC at the RSPV **(a)** at the start of ablation, and **(b)** immediately after ablation.

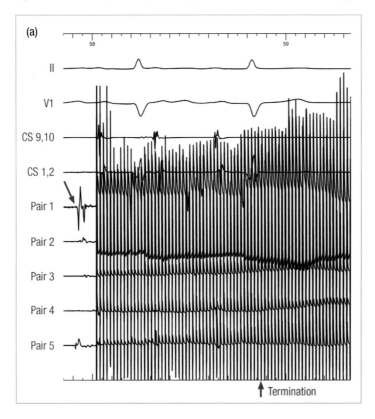

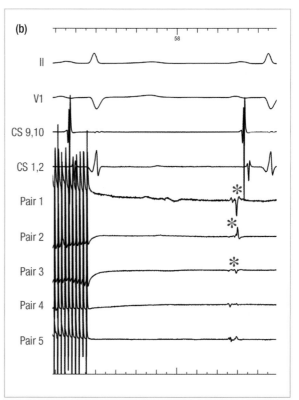

Confirmation of Right Superior Pulmonary Vein Isolation With a Conventional Circular Mapping Catheter

Figure 5 shows the fluoroscopic position of the conventional CMC within the RSPV. In this case (the same as described above), isolation of the RSPV is confirmed using the conventional CMC before and after PVAC mapping and ablation (↓, PV potential eliciting atrial tachycardia; ∗, far-field signal; **Figure 6**).

Figure 6. Confirmation of isolation of the RSPV using the conventional CMC (a) at baseline, and (b) after RF ablation.

Figure 5. Position of the conventional CMC for verification of isolation.

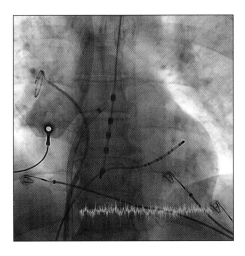

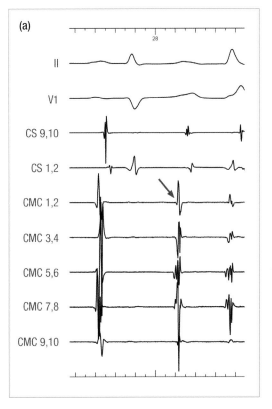

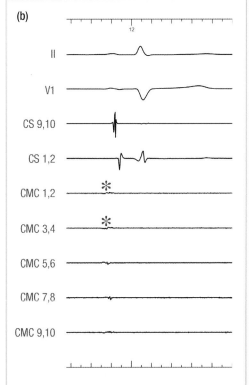

Mapping of Unidirectional Block Using the PVAC

Figure 7 shows a bipolar electrogram recorded with the PVAC within the right inferior pulmonary vein (RIPV) after delivery of RF energy ablation.

The surface electrogram reveals sinus rhythm, a short-coupled atrial ectopic beat (beat 2), and a late atrial ectopic beat (beat 5). The PVAC electrograms indicate entrance block during sinus beats (beats 1, 3, 4, and 6). An idio-PV rhythm (with a cycle length of 2,600 msec) is observed within the RIPV (↓, pairs 3 and 4). This idio-PV rhythm conducts towards the LA (exit conduction) resulting in atrial ectopic beats (∗, beats 2 and 5). Ablation was continued until exit block. Entrance block with exit conduction is an example of unidirectional LA-PV block.

Figure 7. PVAC mapping within the RIPV after RF energy ablation.

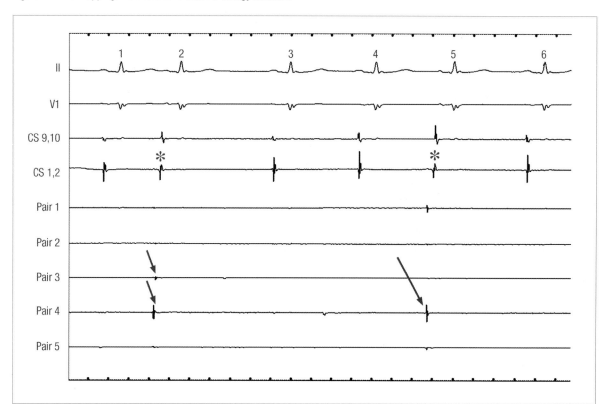

Mapping and Ablation of Atrial Fibrillation Originating from the Superior Vena Cava Using the PVAC

Figure 8 shows the fluoroscopic position of the PVAC at the ostium of the SVC.

Initiation of atrial fibrillation (AF) was observed during administration of adenosine (**Figure 9**). At the start of AF the SVC signals (↓, pair 1) clearly precede CS activation (from CSP to CSD). During the subsequent AF beats, the AF cycle length at the SVC is markedly shortened (±100 msec).

Figure 8. Fluoroscopic position of the PVAC within the SVC. (a) Left anterior oblique (LAO) and (b) right anterior oblique (RAO) views.

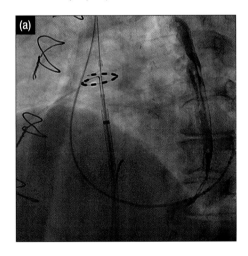
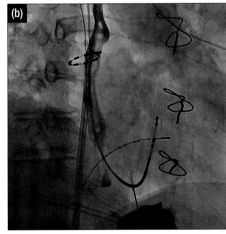

Figure 9. Initiation of AF was observed during administration of adenosine.

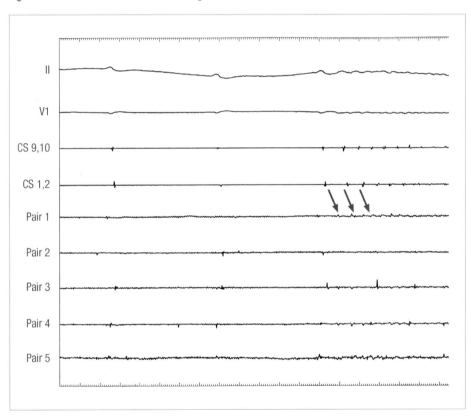

500 msec

In this case (the same as described above), there is distal PVAC mapping within the SVC during sinus rhythm, before and after proximal ablation. Before RF ablation, mapping with PVAC revealed sharp, multiple SVC potentials (↓; **Figure 10a**). After RF energy ablation (1-min application), PVAC mapping revealed electrical isolation of the SVC (**Figure 10b**).

Figure 10. Confirmation of isolation of the SVC with the PVAC (a) at baseline, and (b) after RF energy ablation.

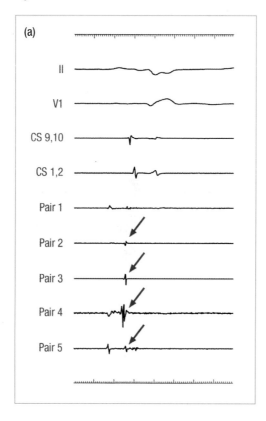
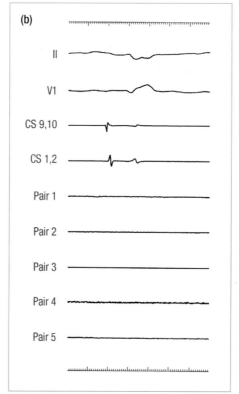

Vagal Response Elicited During Ablation Using the PVAC

PVAC ablation was performed at the LSPV (**Figure 11**).

Prior to the first application, the patient was sedated with a combination of fentanyl and diazepam administered intravenously. The patient showed no signs of pain during ablation. During the application sinus rhythm initially continued with frequent ectopic activity. After 10 sec (**Figure 12**), there was complete asystole for a prolonged period of time after which the application was stopped and CS pacing was performed.

Figure 11. PVAC ablation at the LSPV. (a) Selective PV angiography of the LSPV (LAO), and (b) position of the PVAC (also LAO view).

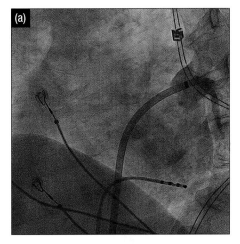 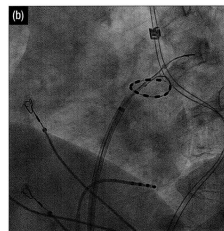

Such a vagal response can be observed in patients under general anesthesia, under conscious sedation, or even in those without any sedation. It is not directly linked to a sensation of pain, and can sometimes occur at the start of the application before there is a significant temperature rise.

Figure 12. Vagal response during PVAC ablation.

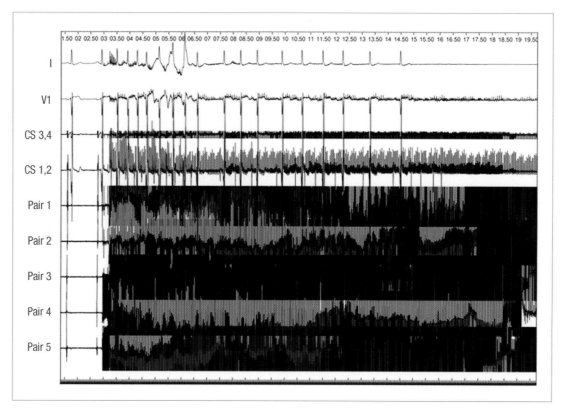

100 msec

Conclusion

- Triggering PVs or non-PV foci can be mapped and ablated with the PVAC

- The PVAC can identify entrance block with exit conduction

- PVAC ablation can elicit vagal responses

Recommended Reading

Arentz T, Macle L, Kalusche D, et al. "Dormant" pulmonary vein conduction revealed by adenosine after ostial radiofrequency catheter ablation. *J Cardiovasc Electrophysiol* 2004;15:1041–7.

Boersma L, Wijffels M, Oral H, et al. Pulmonary vein isolation by duty-cycled bipolar and unipolar radiofrequency energy with a multielectrode ablation catheter. *Heart Rhythm* 2008;5:1635–42.

Boersma LVA, Wijffels MC, Wever EFD, et al. Acute results of PV antrum ablation by a novel circumlinear decapolar catheter with low power duty-cycled RF energy. *Heart Rhythm* 2008;5(Suppl):S368–69 [PO6-32].

Boersma L, Mulder A, Jansen W, et al. Voltage analysis after multi-electrode ablation with duty-cycled bipolar and unipolar radiofrequency energy: a case report. *Europace* 2009;11:1546–8.

Duytschaever M, Anne W, Papiashvili G, et al. Mapping and isolation of the pulmonary veins using the PVAC catheter. *Pacing Clin Electrophysiol* 2010;33:168–78.

Gerstenfeld EP, Dixit S, Callans D, et al. Utility of exit block for identifying electrical isolation of the pulmonary veins. *J Cardiovasc Electrophysiol* 2002;13:971–9.

Hachiya H, Hirao K, Takahashi A, et al. Clinical implications of reconnection between the left atrium and isolated pulmonary veins provoked by adenosine triphosphate after extensive encircling pulmonary vein isolation. *J Cardiovasc Electrophysiol* 2007;18:392–8.

Haïssaguerre M, Jaïs P, Shah DC, et al. Spontaneous initiation of atrial fibrillation by ectopic beats originating in the pulmonary veins. *N Engl J Med* 1998;339:659–66.

Hsieh MH, Tai CT, Lee SH, et al. The different mechanisms between late and very late recurrences of atrial fibrillation in patients undergoing a repeated catheter ablation. *J Cardiovasc Electrophysiol* 2006;17:231–5.

Jaïs P, Hocini M, Macle L, et al. Distinctive electrophysiological properties of pulmonary veins in patients with atrial fibrillation. *Circulation* 2002;106:2479–85.

Lerman BB, Belardinelli L. Cardiac electrophysiology of adenosine. Basic and clinical concepts. *Circulation* 1991;83:1499–509.

Matsuo S, Yamane T, Date T, et al. Reduction of AF recurrence after pulmonary vein isolation by eliminating ATP-induced transient venous re-conduction. *J Cardiovasc Electrophysiol* 2007;18:704–8.

Michaud GF, Martin DT, John RM, et al. Safety using novel multi-array catheters and phased radiofrequency energy in left atrial ablation for persistent atrial fibrillation. *Heart Rhythm* 2008;5(Suppl):S313–14 [PO5-17].

Scharf C, Sneider M, Case I, et al. Anatomy of the pulmonary veins in patients with atrial fibrillation and effects of segmental ostial ablation analyzed by computed tomography. *J Cardiovasc Electrophysiol* 2003;14:150–5.

Scharf C, Boersma L, Davies W, et al. Ablation of persistent atrial fibrillation using multielectrode catheters and duty-cycled radiofrequency energy. *J Am Coll Cardiol* 2009;54:1450–6.

Shah D, Haïssaguerre M, Takahashi A, et al. Differential pacing for distinguishing block from persistent conduction through an ablation line. *Circulation* 2000;102:1517–22.

Shah D, Burri H, Sunthorn H, et al. Identifying far-field superior vena cava potentials within the right superior pulmonary vein. *Heart Rhythm* 2006;3:898–902.

Tang M, Gerds-Li J-H, Nedios S, et al. Optimal fluoroscopic projections for angiographic imaging of the pulmonary vein ostia: lessons learned from the intraprocedural reconstruction of the left atrium and pulmonary veins. *Europace* 2010;12:37–44.

Tritto M, De Ponti R, Salerno-Uriarte JA, et al. Adenosine restores atrio-venous conduction after apparently successful ostial isolation of the pulmonary veins. *Eur Heart J* 2004;25:2155–63.

Van Belle Y, Janse P, Rivero-Ayerza MJ, et al. Pulmonary vein isolation using an occluding cryoballoon for circumferential ablation: feasibility, complications, and short-term outcome. *Eur Heart J* 2007;28:2231–7.

Wieczorek M, Hoeltgen R, Brueck M, et al. Pulmonary vein isolation by dutycycled bipolar and unipolar antrum ablation using a novel multielectrode ablation catheter system: first clinical results. *J Interv Card Electrophysiol* 2010;27:23–31.

Wijffels M, van Oosterhout M, Boersma L, et al. Characterization of *in vitro* and *in vivo* lesions made by a novel multichannel ablation generator and a circumlinear decapolar ablation catheter. *J Cardiovasc Electrophysiol* 2009;20:1142–8.

Abbreviations

AF	atrial fibrillation	**LIPV**	left inferior pulmonary vein
AV	atrioventricular	**LSPV**	left superior pulmonary vein
Bip EGM	bipolar electrogram	**PV**	pulmonary vein
CMC	circular mapping catheter	**PVAC**	Pulmonary Vein Ablation Catheter
CS	coronary sinus	**RA**	right atrium
CSD	distal coronary sinus	**RAO**	right anterior oblique
CSP	proximal coronary sinus	**RF energy**	radiofrequency energy
CT	computed tomography	**RIPV**	right inferior pulmonary vein
IVC	inferior vena cava	**RMPV**	right middle pulmonary vein
LA	left atrium	**RSPV**	right superior pulmonary vein
LAA	left atrial appendage	**Stim-A interval**	stimulus-to-atrium interval
LAO	left anterior oblique	**SVC**	superior vena cava
LA-PV	left atrial pulmonary vein	**Uni EGM**	unipolar electrogram

Index